GW00649798

your health is your wealth

Jacqueline Harvey

HAY HOUSE

Australia • Canada • Hong Kong • India
South Africa • United Kingdom • United States

First published and distributed in the United Kingdom by:
Hay House UK Ltd, 292B Kensal Rd, London W10 5BE. Tel.: (44) 20 8962 1230;
Fax: (44) 20 8962 1239. www.hayhouse.co.uk

Published and distributed in the United States of America by:
Hay House, Inc., PO Box 5100, Carlsbad, CA 92018-5100. Tel.: (1) 760 431 7695 or
(800) 654 5126; Fax: (1) 760 431 6948 or (800) 650 5115. www.hayhouse.com

Published and distributed in Australia by:
Hay House Australia Ltd, 18/36 Ralph St, Alexandria NSW 2015. Tel.: (61) 2 9669 4299;
Fax: (61) 2 9669 4144. www.hayhouse.com.au

Published and distributed in the Republic of South Africa by:
Hay House SA (Pty), Ltd, PO Box 990, Witkoppen 2068. Tel./Fax: (27) 11 467 8904.
www.hayhouse.co.za

Published and distributed in India by:
Hay House Publishers India, Muskaan Complex, Plot No.3, B-2, Vasant Kunj,
New Delhi – 110 070. Tel.: (91) 11 4176 1620; Fax: (91) 11 4176 1630. www.hayhouse.co.in

Distributed in Canada by:
Raincoast, 9050 Shaughnessy St, Vancouver, BC V6P 6E5.
Tel.: (1) 604 323 7100; Fax: (1) 604 323 2600

© Jacqueline Harvey, 2008

The moral rights of the author have been asserted.

All rights reserved. No part of this book may be reproduced by any mechanical, photographic or
electronic process, or in the form of a phonographic recording; nor may it be stored in a retrieval
system, transmitted or otherwise be copied for public or private use, other than for 'fair use'
as brief quotations embodied in articles and reviews, without prior written permission of the
publisher.

The author of this book does not dispense medical advice or prescribe the use of any technique
as a form of treatment for physical or medical problems without the advice of a physician, either
directly or indirectly. The intent of the author is only to offer information of a general nature
to help you in your quest for emotional and spiritual wellbeing. In the event you use any of
the information in this book for yourself, which is your constitutional right, the author and the
publisher assume no responsibility for your actions.

A catalogue record for this book is available from the British Library.

ISBN 978-1-4019-1628-2

Internal photos © Fiona Sheward

Printed in the UK by CPI William Clowes Beccles NR34 7TL

your health is your wealth

Contents

Introduction

It's no surprise that many people are confused about how to lead a healthier life. The media bombard us with conflicting and confusing information on a daily basis, interfering with our ability to have a clear picture about what we need to become fit and well. We've gone from high-carbohydrate diets to low, from low-fat diets to 'good fats' diets (in the form of oily fish, nuts and seeds), and finally from yoga and Pilates to good old-fashioned exercise and sport-based movement.

From one day to the next, the parameters for health change, depending on consumer markets – up until the 26th December everyone is encouraged to eat high-fat and diabetes-producing levels of sugar, all washed down with brain-frying amounts of alcohol – all in the name of Christmas fun! Yet barely a week later we are attacked with a zillion messages from the government and the diet and fitness industries, telling us to lose weight because we're all too fat!

The result is that many people remain uninformed about simple, healthy guidelines about eating and exercise. As recently as September 2007, the Food Standards Agency Survey reported that substantial numbers of Britons still do not understand how to follow a balanced diet despite numerous campaigns such as '5 a day', highlighting which foods are healthy or not. People are unsure how much bread and pasta they should eat, the key role played by fruit and vegetables, and even how much damage products high in fat or sugar can do to their health. Officials were disappointed that so many of the 2,094 people questioned across the UK gave incorrect answers – 42 per cent did not know that we should only eat high-fat or high-sugar foods occasionally!

It deeply concerns me that so many people would ignore the government's advice and choose instead to look to faddish celebrity diets for help. Poor diets kill 69,400 Britons every year – ten per cent of all deaths. Of these, 42,200 are linked to a lack of fruit and vegetables, 20,200 are due to excess salt, 3,500 to an intake of saturated fats and 3,500 to excessive sugar.

My aim is to demystify the process by giving you the information you need, not only to change your body but to have a positive impact on your mental and emotional health. Along the way, I've discovered that our health story is more complex than I had imagined.

To help ourselves, we have to take on board (now more than at any other time) that being fit and healthy requires a little more effort than simply going off to the gym or pool, or indeed taking a quick stroll in the park a few times a week. Managing our health must now include monitoring our food intake, regular exercise and effective mind management. These three elements work together in a symbiotic way to create a healthy body.

Health is about what we eat, how we move, and what we think and feel. Neglecting any of these three areas will compromise your health – so information on just eating, exercise or mental development does not address the whole picture of your health.

AN EMBARRASSMENT OF RICHES?

Our society has changed so much – most Western economies have an abundance of material wealth, unprecedented in previous eras. And yet this very wealth is compromising our health – we suffer a growing number of preventable illnesses and disorders. Obesity, heart disease, high blood pressure, diabetes and a plethora of stress-related ailments affect our health and the quality of our lives. All these illnesses can be improved or even healed with healthy eating, exercise and positive mind management.

The poor health of our nation has its roots in the fact that we have lost our own innate knowledge of how to be and remain healthy. The focus has been on intellectual and material advancement, at the cost of our physical, emotional and spiritual health. Our 'abundant' lifestyle has not made us happier or more well-balanced; in fact, the reverse is true, and on the rise: we are becoming unhealthy due to our wealth.

The three-step plan detailed in this book stems from research I've carried out throughout my life, which has led me to a career which, even as recently as 20 years ago, did not exist. I spent much of my early life suffering from various illnesses, due to a lack of knowledge about what my body needed to function in a healthy way. Over the years, thanks to a thorough education about myself and how my body works, these ailments have been healed or, if not, I've got them under control. But they played a major role in my efforts to understand the link between mind and body. Subsequently, through years of research and work as a holistic personal fitness trainer, I have developed a lifestyle system that not only maintains health and fitness but which, as an added bonus, has contributed to my spiritual enrichment and personal growth.

By choosing to prioritize your body, you choose to rekindle an ancient bond, deep within you that, ultimately, allows for greater overall health.

Unhappiness affects how we think and what we can manifest in all areas of our lives. Currently some 300,000 under-35s in the UK claim Incapacity Benefit due to mental and behavioural disorders. Our prescription drug use is currently running in the region of £31 million a year. Do these figures reflect a happy, healthy or wealthy nation?

A recent study from the University of Newcastle in Australia looked at the effect of materialism on mental health. The result? Excessive materialism has a bad effect on mental health: 'Possession of conspicuous goods is associated neither with global life satisfaction, psychological health nor with a love of life.'[1]

Your Health Is Your Wealth offers a lifestyle system for developing greater personal growth through positive nutrition, exercise and relaxation techniques. We have to look beyond the basic materials of life to become wealthy in the future, because to fully experience all the riches life has to offer, we need our health. A life tainted and restricted by pain, mobility problems or other forms of ill health is only partially lived.

This book aims to redress the balance. It is essential that we are not short-sighted about our bodies and adopt healthier living habits because, with age, conditions like high blood pressure and arthritis, although not life-threatening, deplete our physical, emotional and even financial resources. A fragmented person cannot be fully productive or at ease with life.

Chapter 1 explains how we have become 'disembodied' and how we can correct this with lifestyle changes that promote a more balanced existence. I've called this chapter 'The Big Picture' because in it I try to provide an overview of the theory behind the practice of good health.

Chapter 2 looks at how stretching and meditation exercises can combat both the physical and mental effects of stress. By using these techniques and practices I hope you will gain the freedom and growth that my clients and I have experienced, and that will enrich the quality of your life.

Chapter 3 investigates the confusing issues relating to food and whether it really is nourishment or poison, concluding with a practical guide of how to eat in a way that maintains health without removing the pleasure to be had from good food.

The benefits of exercise and how it affects your mental health are the focus of Chapter 4. I have not felt it necessary to consider the routine aspects of exercise such as how many sit-ups, bench-presses or miles should be performed to become fit, because that is a totally individual decision that needs to be assessed each time exercise is performed. However, at the end of the book are some suggestions on how to get started on a movement programme. I have tried to give you the information you need to assess why you should do weight-bearing exercise, and what happens in the body and mind that makes these movements so essential to life.

Investment in our health is essential if we are to reap the benefits now and later in life.

In the future we will all have to become more responsible for our healthcare as the British government looks at extending the age of retirement – we are going to have to work far longer than our parents did. And, because the NHS is so under-funded, it will no longer operate in its existing form when we do finally retire.

For this reason and so many others, true health – a sound mind in a sound body – should be everyone's goal, and *Your Health Is Your Wealth* can show you just how achievable this goal is.

Chapter 1

The Big Picture

We are obsessed with our bodies today – how they look, feel and the sensations they give us – it's almost as if we are trying to reclaim our skin. Few of us are satisfied with either the shape we're in or the future health of our nation. A high level of anxiety and confusion surrounds our feelings about our bodies. I think this anxiety and confusion have come about as an effect of our material development.

As part of our history as a civilization we have lost the ability to feel at ease with ourselves; our bodies have become vehicles solely for the mind. This shift left our culture with no language or practical philosophy that unifies mind and body. The result is that the majority of us feel alienated within ourselves, lacking in real energy and prone to modern-day illnesses which undermine our health.

In this chapter I'll take a look at how certain historical factors supported this separation. I feel that an alternative way of handling our lives – through the triad of exercise, movement and state of mind – is the key to a united, healthier self. I have found these three components to be the basis for 'whole body' communication and health.

FRAGMENTED BODIES

In Western society our inability to hear our bodies speak to us is no accident. A view of the body as separate from the mind, two components existing in detached realms, is part of our social history and the result of a limited and partial education. When scientific thought became the dominant knowledge base, this was the inevitable result.

The 'mind–body' separation began, I believe, in the 18th century – the so-called 'Age of Enlightenment'. Part of the new emphasis on scientific discovery involved a new way of viewing the body: as a series of mechanical parts rather than an organic whole.

Our everyday language is littered with this type of thinking; we talk about the body in parts – 'My bum is too big, breasts are too small, nose is too flat, stomach enormous' – all are seen as subject to change with no thought about how these bits contribute to the overall whole. This is why altering selected parts of our bodies with plastic surgery rarely makes anyone happy. The change our spirit is truly craving is a reconnection and development *internally* – achieving this creates a feeling of health and wellbeing, true balance and deep self-esteem.

Pre-Enlightenment European culture advocated a more holistic view precisely because it emphasized spiritual growth. There was no separation between the mind, physical wellbeing and the environment.

Everyday life was seen in 'other-worldly' terms. Existence on the earth was only important as a precursor to the life hereafter. The world was thought to be ruled by forces that could be observed. Mother Nature was perceived as ruling the physical world, which in turn had been made by God.

The universe was understood as made up of interconnected but equal power relationships. The mental sphere, governed by man, and the physical sphere, governed by nature (the feminine), were seen as a comprehensive reality dominated by neither but existing as a symbiotic, mutually beneficial whole.

What was known about the body was rarely viewed without the emotions: a person's relationship to God or their environment influenced who they were. Information on how to feed and maintain health was sought and found in nature. The secret to good health and progress was thought to be held not just in the body but in the land. Nature was a force to be worked with as an equal, not dominated or controlled.

The Ancient Greeks

In ancient Greek culture, the body was seen to play an important role in the development of the whole person. In their book *The Greeks*, Guhl and Koner explain:

> *Exercise was no less an important part of education than the mutual progress itself. The harmonious development of the body was thought to be the basis for attaining self-conscious determination in the practical demands of life. The process of*

acting through means of the body on the mind was practised in the gymnastic and agnostic institutions of Greece.[1]

However, exercise was largely the prerogative of men, and this type of social division relegated women to the role of second-class citizens – a feature that remained part of Western society right up until the late 19th century (and, some would argue, beyond!). For the earliest feminist commentators, nature and women's connection to it only served to enhance the notion of the mind and body being separate entities, with men seen as the 'thinkers' while women were viewed as closer to animals and lacking in the ability to use reason. Women were considered ruled by their bodies, by biology (periods, childbirth, etc.), while men had transcended their bodies through the creation of culture.

World Faiths/The Chakras

Examples of holistic lifestyles are evident in many world faiths, particularly in the East – in the Hindu faith the medical and spiritual system views the body as a network of energy structures called the *chakras*. The notion of the Tree of Life (developed in Judaism) and Taoism in China also integrate body, mind, soul and environment into cultural life.

As in pre-Enlightenment Europe, there is in these philosophies an emphasis on the continuous flow of energy between various points on the body that helps us to know ourselves and our environment. The aim of these practices is to develop knowledge of the physical world for a greater understanding of the mental and spiritual realms, which in turn allow us to catch a glimpse of the wider universe and our place within it.

Many alternative practitioners today still base their therapies on the chakra system's understanding of the body and universe – which in essence consists of seven main energy disks sited at various points on the body. (See figure below)

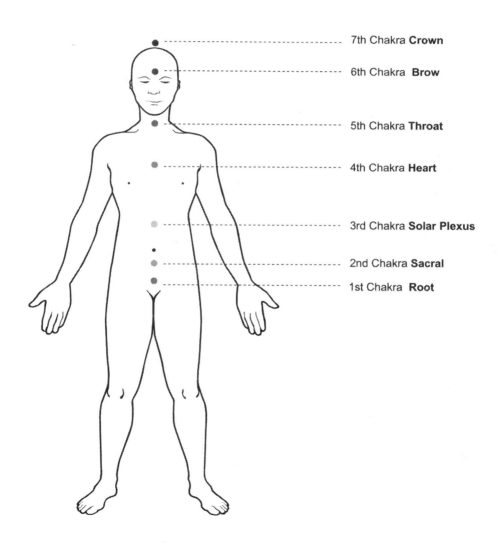

7th Chakra **Crown**

6th Chakra **Brow**

5th Chakra **Throat**

4th Chakra **Heart**

3rd Chakra **Solar Plexus**

2nd Chakra **Sacral**

1st Chakra **Root**

These chakras or free-floating wheels of energy also relate to various elemental forces in the physical world, as the body is nearly always seen as a micro-reflection of the wider material plane. For instance, the first chakra is positioned at the end of the spine and correlates to the earth, while the second chakra, situated in the lower abdomen, relates to the moon.

The seven points in the body are hierarchical – from the lowest form of knowledge to the highest. From this view we can only truly grow in a balanced way if we use knowledge from all points. Learning through thought alone is only partial and one-sided because it is untested in the real material world.

Living a full life without working on our body would be like building a house without foundations. It is vital that life's foundations be clearly set before energy can flow freely between the different levels. And as Chakra One is concerned with the body's general health, material and financial existence, the importance of maintaining a positive environment in which the heart, mind and soul can dwell is thought to be paramount.

There are several positive elements to this life view – and some rather glaring problems. On one level it is great because it teaches us how to relate to our body and the world in a non-superficial way. Also, its advocates do not see physical or material development as mutually exclusive for spiritual development, but rather use these as the basis for higher levels of growth. In reality many of us run into problems, however, when we become stuck on the base level at a time when we should be moving on – this prevents us from acquiring the greater knowledge and experience that exist throughout the higher levels.

The chakra system is not concerned with the *appearance* of health or how good things look on the outside, but forces us to look beyond the surface to see how our whole system works, in order to correct any natural or environmental imbalances. To successfully attain this enlightenment you need to apply discipline, focus and determination via various modes of exercise, meditation and nutritional therapy. It is non-competitive and utterly individual – your journey to self-knowledge and your body is totally unique; along the way, each of us discovers who we are and where our strengths and limitations lie.

Choosing to adopt a healthier lifestyle, to get the maximum out of life, is not viewed as a fad or fashion in Hindu culture; instead it is a necessary act on the path to greater self-awareness. Prevention is always better than cure, and if one achieves true communication between the body and mind, self-diagnosis and healing become possible – you will have the ability to tune into and heal others through your own journey.

I think that one of the challenges of our age is to share our abundance with others. The whole notion of balance and self-empowerment is inherent to the chakra system because it teaches us to become more proactive when we are feeling unstable. With increased self-awareness we can quickly recognize when we're getting stressed due to overwork or emotional problems, then take the appropriate action to alleviate this or soften its effects. If you work hard, then playing hard or planning significant rest will enable you to function at optimum levels for longer.

Essentially the chakra system is about keeping energy flowing through your whole body. If you allow work, for example, to dominate your life for long periods of time, then you run the risk of premature illness. Illness begins when our energy becomes blocked or stuck – this in itself offers us a pretty clear insight into how our modern attitude to material wealth is helping to cause so many modern diseases.

Unlike the spiritual practices of the East, Christianity has been the main spiritual influence in Europe. This faith, coupled with the scientific and industrial revolutions whose seeds were sown during the Enlightenment, helped to confuse how we relate to our bodies.

With the emergence of Christianity, responsibility for our health and access to our own emotional health and the world around us became restricted. Information and knowledge built up from our own experience became devalued because it was outside the Church, which also had political influence with the ruling government of the day. The Crusades and, later, the witch-hunts are examples of how the Church dealt with those who refused to adopt its view of life. These events marked not only a loss of our personal freedoms but also the start of our dependence on the state as a central definer of truth.

According to Richard Sennett, in the Catholic faith there is no system of knowledge that directly links people to their bodies. Rather, the body is viewed as a vessel for the mind, and so can (and often, should) be denied physical pleasures like sex and food (realized in the vows of celibacy and poverty for priests). Believers were expected to endure enormous amounts of pain to reinforce the belief of mind over matter, to illustrate one's belief in the faith. 'The only knowledge that is valuable is that of the spiritual, i.e. of God Himself.'[2]

Christianity in this form requires us to accept that the body, work and our social status are secondary to our spiritual lives, hence we need to pass spiritual tests in order to win or lose salvation. Everyday life turns out to be about enduring pain, suffering and sacrifice in order to find our place with God. Christianity's teachings offer numerous examples of denial, punishment and guilt as well as pain rather than discipline. These negative experiences interrupt all dialogue between the mind and body and distort the way we relate to others in society. The resulting confusion has helped us to feel uncomfortable and even to deny our sensations – yet at the same time we are expected to empathize with the pain of our fellow men. Some of our natural bodily functions, like sex, are seen in negative terms – sex for pleasure rather than procreation is viewed as part of the animal sphere, rather than human, and is therefore something we should feel guilty about.

By the beginning of the 15th century, this confusion and other social inequalities – mainly poverty – led leaders in society to question the belief in God as the divine creator of the universe. Society became disenchanted with the Church and the corruption of its priests. Consequently, by the late 18th century the power of the clergy had disintegrated to a level that allowed for science to emerge as the dominant force.

Disbelief in church authority created a search for autonomous knowledge of the world. Science sought to produce independent truth about life that could be discovered through experimentation to formulate 'laws'. However, this method of creating knowledge about the world served only to reinforce the mind/body split inherited from Christianity, as it gave the mind supremacy over the body.

Our bodies were relegated to second position, seen only as receptors relaying and interpreting what we experience about our environment. It was then left to the mind to decide what was 'real'. No longer was there any room for divine providence, and nature became a force to be dominated to our benefit. The idea of natural, balanced movement between different parts of the whole was sacrificed for a focus on the parts, a much more mechanistic view of life. As Norman Hampson explains,

> Nature instead of being a mere collection of phenomena,
> a hotchpotch of occult influences or canvas on which an
> inscrutable providence painted its mysterious symbols, was a
> system of intelligible forces. God was a mathematician whose
> calculations, although infinite in their subtle complexity, were
> accessible to man's intelligence. What was still unknown could
> eventually be discovered.[3]

To a large extent this agenda still dominates our culture today. This philosophical shift was motivated in part by the need to manipulate the world for human benefit. By raising living standards, we have enjoyed a unique period of security and material wealth. However, many of us today feel ill at ease with the society we have created. We feel displaced, not only environmentally but also in our own bodies.

I agree with those social commentators who suggest that the great emphasis on material wealth has led to the degradation of human relationships, and that the Enlightenment signalled a breakdown in communication. We cannot live like machines, as this leaves us with no language to explain how we feel in ourselves – for science has no place for feelings. Science and the cult of reason and logic have made it increasingly difficult for the feelings that arise from within our bodies to be given any legitimacy, so messages from the body are often relegated to the realm of the imagination. Increasingly people feel isolated, ill at ease physically and alone, even in relationships, searching for what they know to be missing within themselves but cannot put their finger on. Stuck on the external, some seek superficial answers to internal issues like the idea that eternal youth can be bought from the plastic surgeon. Even simple information about how the body works has now become lost in a sea of confusion, diminishing our ability to hear intuitively and understand our own truth, decreasing our ability to create a healthy and truly wealthy life.

One example of such confusion is that it was widely believed over the latter part of the last century that women released only one egg a month from which a pregnancy could occur. From this fact the law of a 'safe' and 'unsafe' time to become pregnant was formed. Doctors happily dismissed reports from women who claimed they became pregnant *after* ovulation. These women were simply labelled medical freaks, liars or ignorant of their own cycles.

Now the medical profession has found, via research, that women can and do ovulate more than once a month, a random process that increases fertility. The 28-day menstrual cycle law that was drummed into young women at school in the 1970s and 80s has been made redundant.

TAKING CONTROL

The price for our alienating our internal selves has been a generalized lack of understanding of our own natural healing processes. With no encouragement to express how we feel, we have become ever more dependent on state-registered medical professionals with vested financial interests in not curing the source of many common ailments.

For example, many women at some point in their lives may have developed a 'yeast' infection for which the doctor invariably prescribes a product that does not cure the problem but only temporarily relieves the symptoms. This product is expensive and most women use it at least once in their lives, generating a small fortune for the pharmaceutical companies who produce it. It is simply not in their financial interests to provide a cure for the symptoms. It is only by chance that some women may find out that this ailment of excessive yeast growth is usually a dietary problem or provoked by commonly used antibiotics.

Ideally, the medical profession should work in a more ethical way by using a combination of nutritional therapy and prescription drugs – this would educate women on how to balance their diets to prevent high yeast growth. More education needs to be available about the effects of antibiotics on the body so that they are used less frequently. This way of treating sickness sets out to cure but also helps create a preventative system that allows *us* to be more active in *our own* healing.

If we look at the area of exercise, only recently have some practitioners accepted the fact that in order to change the body permanently, exercise is not the only factor – we must be prepared to change the way we think and live – hence the term 'lifestyle change'.

I have found that one of most crucial issues to creating change in the body is to accept responsibility for your own health. Working as a personal fitness trainer over the years, some clients have come to me for help in the hope that I would take responsibility for their body. To accept this role would only help to support the very culture of dependence that is so prevalent today. Each of us can only change when we are ready to take control of our own healing. I see my role as the facilitator; my clients are the ones actually in charge. Solving these issues requires a great deal of trust and education about getting them to know how their individual body works, while repeatedly illustrating how their mind and emotions influence this process. Rarely has it been solely concerned with creating the latest 'look'. Clients who feel generally happy with their lives tend to change their bodies more quickly than those struggling with emotional, mental or financial stress.

It takes courage to change any aspect of yourself, and sometimes it is all too easy to blame someone else. Employing a trainer three times a week is not the end of the problem but really the start of a long journey into self-discovery. Choosing to change from inside will cause changes externally, but this takes time – an increasingly rare commodity in our time-poor culture. If we accept responsibility for our bodies, then we will make the time for ourselves. Exercise, for instance, can be seen as a form of active meditation where you can calm the mind and place positive thoughts in your head about how to live in a better way. Movement cleanses not just the body but also the mind, ridding it of unhelpful thoughts.

Yes, science is a truly awesome system of knowledge, but the notion that the human body and thoughts are the same as the workings of a computer is just plain wrong. In the fields of medicine and sport, scientists have repeatedly had to concede that what they thought to be true is not, because their 'data' do not take into account the complexity of the human mind, body and emotions. We need to develop a language that reflects this dynamic process rather than presenting us with ultimate 'truths'.

The answer to why people do not have a positive working relationship with their bodies can only be understood by looking at Western economic and social development. Our present society values material wealth above all else. As I've mentioned, Eastern societies and even our own past gave equal balance to the body, mind and spirit. It's a link that each of us truly needs and desires.

I am not advocating a return to the past, nor promoting alternative medicine. I would prefer to see an *integrated* system that encourages health and fitness as essential parts of life. In acquiring self-knowledge we are tapping into an unending stream of wealth – few of us ever realize our full potential. Illnesses, both physical and mental, are clear indicators that we should start to prioritize our health. What's the good of money if you're ill? Sports science, nutritional therapy, naturopathy, chiropractic, acupuncture and traditional medicine can all be used together, as they all have a part to play in producing knowledge about the body and, therefore, long-term health. No one system has all the answers, but each has something to add in the quest to find out about ourselves.

I believe, like many holistic practitioners and Eastern mystics, that self-knowledge through the body is the foundation and primal centre for a greater understanding of others and the world. Once we know ourselves, our lives become more within our control. We gain the ability to discriminate between what is real and what is only illusion so that we make decisions that will increase our personal health and wealth.

THE STAR OF WEALTH

The Star of Wealth is the key to harnessing your own inner resources to improve and increase your health on all levels. By becoming active, eating well and taking control of your mind, you will have a realistic, integrated lifestyle that allows you to reconnect your body to your mind. Not only will you increase your ability to hear your own voice but you will also have control over your wellbeing and the strength to direct your life – your very own personalized system for total health.

Figures 2 and 3 illustrate how the two triangles work together to form the six-pointed Star of Wealth. Each point on the star is integral to the achievement of your own total health picture.

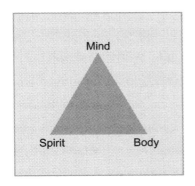

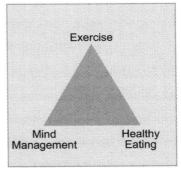

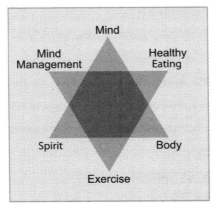

EXERCISE, NUTRITION AND STATE OF MIND

Whenever we talk about exercise, the focus seems to be on how little we do, and our discussions are littered with guilty anecdotes. Usually, at some point in the conversation, friends, relatives or indeed clients will look to me for some sort of absolution from their self-inflicted 'sin'. My tactful response has always been to say, 'Just start to do something and you will feel better.' Most of us know inherently that this is true – we need to move around to be healthy.

All living organic matter is in a state of constant movement and flow. We all have our own individual and innate pattern of growth and change, which is made up of periods of activity interspersed with rest. Non-movement is to resist this flow of natural energy, which disconnects internally and results in blockages or decay – our total development is dependant on this cycle.

Movement is reflexive action that occurs in the body from birth until death, which we can influence either positively or negatively by the way in which we care for ourselves – how we choose to live will improve or decrease the flow of energy.

For instance, if we look at our early growth cycle it shows the important role movement plays in helping us to become adults. A baby has a predetermined cycle of growth that is a balance of feeding, movement and rest – it will start with learning how to crawl, then how to walk and finally how to run. This sequence of physical activity enables an infant's body to develop into that of a child, a teenager, then finally an adult, coupled with an enormous volume of mental stimulation about their new environment.

However, in our culture this growth cycle stops by the time we reach our teens: it is only up until then that we are guided and encouraged to grow in this whole and natural way. After that, we alone become responsible for our health and physical maintenance, as adults, and as our education regarding this area is still only in its infancy, looking after ourselves in this way dramatically declines. Unless we participate in sport, no programme of further education about the dynamic nature of our bodies is taught in the UK, and yet this is intrinsic to our quality of life.

Parents, schools and the state have only just started to prioritize health and exercise because of the vast increase in preventable illness, which affects our wealth as individuals and as a nation – we live in a culture that grossly underestimates the value of exercise even though it enriches our bodies and empowers our minds.

As today's teenagers grow into adulthood, the bliss of life without guidance creates a slowed or non-moving body that paves the way for stagnation, which can later form the type of blockages that contribute to our ever-increasing health problems. High blood pressure, heart attacks, obesity, strokes, diabetes and cancer are now the norm in progressively younger populations.

If we spend our lives seeking status, money, love and experience, there is little time left over to nurture our bodies. It is surprising that more people do not alter their lifestyles given the avalanche of warning signals like chronic fatigue, aches and pains that afflict so many of us – in fact, we are so accustomed to disregarding our body that we ignore its cries to stop, slow down or rest.

Most people begin to wonder where it all went wrong when finally the pressure cooker blows and we no longer have the freedom to move around or perform in the way we want – high blood pressure, diabetes and obesity all curb our life experience.

Within our bodies, the heart clearly reflects the principle of movement. A healthy heart continually pumps blood around the body with periods of rest at night when it beats more slowly. If it becomes blocked or fails to beat, we die or, at the very least, our lives become restricted by enforced drug, food and exercise regimes.

All cell renewal, major organ function and detoxification rely on the heart's ability to pump blood around the body. But the heart itself cannot be reduced to a part or function; it can only be considered as integral to the whole. We need to stop thinking of exercise as a special event or 'treat', beneficial only to our bodies, and look at how it benefits our mind and emotions.

We cannot expect our mind to function effectively if our bodies are not fully nurtured. We need to look at ourselves in a holistic way – our actions and thoughts affect our bodies, personal relationships and environment. Instead of remaining fixed on constantly trying to raise living standards, we actually need to broaden the quality of our life experience – de-stress, and spend more time with ourselves to rest, detox or regenerate. Like the heart, if we become blocked, we become disconnected from our true needs, and emotionally depressed by a lack of stimulation, which impairs our understanding of the world.

Nutrition and Exercise

Eating nutritious food is vital to both our physical and mental output and growth – it holds exercise and state-of-mind techniques together, though all are equally important and necessary for total health. Poor nutrition in early life has been proven to stunt both physical growth and mental function – which can lead to diminished earning power and lack of true fulfilment in life.

Your body is an orb of specific information about you – your past, present and future – so it makes sense to be mindful of what you give it to eat. Food is not your enemy.

When we don't discriminate about what we eat, though, our bodies reject certain foods in order to ensure that it is truly being fed – eating poor-quality food only encourages us to feel weak and ill. In fact, many substances sold to us as 'food' have little right to the title. They in no way contribute to our bodies' health and have poor nutritional value – junk food and processed products fall into this category.

Doctors, nutritionists and health professionals now agree that many ailments and diseases that plague our culture are food-related, which is another way of saying that they are *preventable*. Recent studies into the importance for school children of eating breakfast, how certain foods aid brainpower, and the effects of high alcohol intake, all give us an insight into the importance of food. But this is only the tip of the iceberg. If we balance the food we eat with exercise and relaxation, our mental output increases and stress levels are reduced.

Energy and food are inextricably linked – if we are constantly preoccupied with finding our next meal or we are 'out of fuel', we would achieve very little materially, living at the mercy of our biology. While thankfully most people in our society have moved on from this, we've now created a situation where *too much* energy is being placed in our bodies. Without the balance of exercise to use up the excess energy, the result can be obesity and illnesses such as metabolic syndrome and heart disease.

All of our organs are part of the greater whole of our being, and each is of equal status. There is no reason why conventional medicine – which, after forceful wranglings with alternative practitioners, is finally adopting a more holistic view of health – shouldn't be able to help. Our bodies should not necessarily be dissected – split into parts that operate independently – with the mind as the governing agent. More and more, the evidence proves that our minds and our emotions greatly influence our physical health.

Naturopaths and other holistic practitioners have long argued that, as all parts of the body are in equilibrium, treatments for ailments must take into account the *whole* system in order to treat the underlying causes and not just the symptoms of illness. If you apply these principles to the field of exercise, the route to weight loss will clearly not only involve more movement but also include changing the way you eat, and even the way you think, to achieve long-lasting results.

For weight loss, we need to assess your total body fat-to-muscle ratio, introduce a healthy dietary plan that reduces fat and calorie intake, and then create a workout plan to increase how much energy you burn. And this should be combined with a total lifestyle plan to help you put the programme into action – a plan that would include 'mind-management' techniques to help you get rid of poor habits and cultivate new, more positive ones.

The typical pear shape is partly biology but can be improved with exercise – we spend too much time seated at a computer, on the telephone, or watching the television, a position that causes the energy in our lower bodies to slow down and store excess fat. Meanwhile our upper body shrinks from lack of exercise.

One of our greatest challenges with food today is to find the balance between eating for pleasure (living to eat) and eating for the best nutrition (eating to live). I believe that having a better understanding of what you're eating and why, combined with exercise, helps you to achieve a balance that will keep you healthy.

State of Mind

We feel guilty and lazy if we are not constantly in pursuit of something or someone. This quest to accumulate more and more has created an artificial speed that our bodies find difficult to cope with. Another name for this? Stress. Other parts of the world do not focus on amassing wealth as a life journey like we do in the West, and as a result they have a slower way of life – one that we only glimpse when we're there on holiday!

Abroad it's so easy to spot freshly arrived Brits – they're the ones who look like they're on 'speed', wanting to cram as much as possible into their two weeks of so-called 'rest'.

Without adequate physical and mental rest, our minds cannot recharge, they become stuck in monotone thought patterns and we find we can't think outside the box or escape from the prison of our own making. And while our bodies might just be able to carry on in repetitive tasks or lifestyles, our minds need more colour, texture and, some would say, stimulation to grow. Active rest and mind management – through meditation, visualization and affirmations – allow for regeneration by removing the mundane and putting us back into our bodies, helping to keep us grounded and focused.

Exercise on its own is not as beneficial as when it is complemented, balanced out, with proper mental, physical and emotional rest. Exercise and rest form a symbiotic bond that lengthens our progression or growth – we all know people who have suffered from burn-out due to inadequate rest, thereby prematurely reducing their output. Your body and your life need time to cleanse and heal to boost your ability to flow – it is essential to your mental and spiritual health.

I aim to reduce the level of confusion surrounding personal fitness, nutrition and mind management in the following chapters, so that you'll have the foundation and tools necessary to know yourself better and take control of your total health.

Chapter 2
Reclaiming Your Health

MIND WORKS

While we have to take on board our history to understand its impact on our present health situation, I feel the time is right, now, for us to move forward by taking responsibility for ourselves to shape our own lives. Your health, happiness and general prosperity lie in your ability to work at optimum levels – this can only be made possible by looking after all of the parts that make up the whole you: body, mind and soul.

For me this process begins with the mind (the uppermost point of the Star of Wealth), because without the right attitude and intentions to achieve our goals, we usually end up sabotaging our own efforts.

The mind constantly interacts with and responds to the needs of the body – so, if you're going to change and improve your health and indeed your life, you have to change the way you think. How can you achieve long-term success if you don't really think you deserve it!

Later on in Chapter 4, I will talk about situations that block us from exercising, but the single most significant (and overriding) factor that hinders progress (apart from physical disability) has to be negative thinking. Self-doubt, poor self-belief and a pessimistic attitude towards our bodies are all expressions of a communication breakdown within us. Feeling ashamed or guilty, we really do not expect our bodies to react positively to the stimulation of exercise or to eating a truly nutritious diet – I've seen clients refuse to perform the most basic routines, become verbally abusive or repeatedly miss appointments because they feel so negative about themselves.

I believe these feelings are rooted deep within many of us. The answer isn't to ignore them or suppress them, but to acknowledge them so they can be dealt with positively. One way of doing this is by building confidence and thinking positively about all we do and say – it's a challenging but very effective method of preparing for success and overcoming obstacles, disappointments and delays. An optimistic but realistic attitude helps to 'reset' our minds and get rid of all those unhelpful thought patterns that can stop us acting constructively. Without making it too much of a chore, we need to let go of and deal with mental baggage that prevents us taking positive steps towards change in our lives.

Here are some tips to help you boost your confidence about changing your body:

- If you find your mind drifting into negative dialogue, join in the conversation and consciously talk back aloud and correct the statements, so that 'I'll never get be slim' changes to 'I know I can make myself fit and healthy.' Or 'Why am I doing this to myself? I feel so tired and want to stop!' to 'This is good for me – I just need to relax into it!' Always cancel a negative with an affirmative and eventually the pessimism will die as you no longer feed it.

- Be clear about what you want to achieve – you will only produce a fuzzy outcome if you cannot pinpoint a clear goal. You may need to set short-term goals that will eventually help you to achieve your long-term aim. For example, if you want to eat more healthily, overhauling your whole diet might be difficult to cope with, but if you take out one type of poor-quality food per week, over the course of a few months your eating habits will have considerably improved.

- Research and plan a realistic route to achieving this goal – it's pointless setting a goal like running 10km with little to no preparation, as you'll fail and blame your body. Give yourself the best possible chance of success by preparing with shorter runs leading up to 10km over a few months or so.

- Record and chart your progress – seeing change will help to inspire you to keep on-track; also you'll easily see when you're going off-track. Likewise, if your goal has been reached quickly, don't remain in your comfort zone – move forward while the going is good.

- If, for whatever reason, you don't hit your target, do not beat yourself up about it, as this will only delay your ability to move forward again. Life is full of unknown obstacles, so temper disappointment with helpful self-talk like 'I did the best I could' or 'I can always try to improve a bit later on.'

- If at first you don't succeed, try, try and try again! Perseverance is key to change, because without continuous effort you will not maintain the changes you've created, let alone meet your target.

- You will need support and inspiration to keep you on-track, so seek inspiration from people or friends who want to achieve or have similar goals to yours – they will help to keep you motivated.

- Visualize and affirm how you would like to change your body or lifestyle. Think about it before you go to bed at night – having a clear picture in your subconscious of how you would like to be will help to support and recreate that image in reality.

My sessions with clients are dominated by coaching, positive thinking and verbalizing, and I repeatedly get them to do what is right for their individual bodies so that the magic of long-lasting change occurs.

Once clients see what they can achieve, it builds their confidence and a greater trust in all the processes that make up the Star of Wealth.

Like most activities, your mind can be retrained to experience or view changes in a positive way so that, for example, the more regular exercise you take, the less mental resistance there is to the processes. And the easier exercise becomes, the more likely it is to produce pleasurable and uplifting thoughts to do with life issues and problem solving because you will be more relaxed.

Whether this is due to chemical secretions in the body, the effect of using relaxing music to accompany movement, or simply a reduction in stress levels brought about by an increased flow of oxygen to the brain, those who exercise regularly find they *need* it in their lives for their brains to function at their best.

Exercise is a mind-management tool – while moving, your mind works with your body in a unified way. You're granted valuable 'me time', where your mind is free to create mental patterns and clear out the constant chatter that keeps you from hearing yourself. Structured movement behaves in a dynamic way – we need this extra time and space to think away from our all-too-congested lives.

Over the years, the changes I've noticed in clients' personalities have been some of the most rewarding life experiences for me as a trainer – to see people become happier, more confident and taking control of their lives is joyous. Through this empowerment many take a more active role in their communities by forming new friendships and widening their social network, as well as changing their views on what they can really achieve in other areas of their lives. They have learned that it takes strength and courage to change – attributes they have brought from within themselves to achieve success. And even if they don't always succeed, they know that they have the skills, know-how and inner resources to put things right.

STRESS: CAUSES AND EFFECTS

Everyone will agree that our everyday lives have become too stressful. Stress compromises the way we should live and impairs our judgement – we accept stress as part of how we now live, but it interferes with both our health and our happiness. Prolonged stress is not good for us because it lessens our ability to deal with life's challenges, making us vulnerable to illness and poor judgement.

I am a firm believer that you can reduce your everyday stress levels by understanding what is going on inside your head and body.

We need to be aware of the harmful effect stress hormones have – making their presence felt in ailments such as IBS, migraines, obesity, high blood pressure, heart disease, etc. Stress-release techniques should be an essential part of your daily health regime alongside eating right and exercising. Managing stress allows you to experience life in a more harmonious way, free from anxiety and, therefore, better equipped to deal with any obstacles that come your way.

The Environment

In Chapter 3 we'll look at why it's important to eat the best quality food you can, but I would like to emphasize here just how food sprayed with chemicals affects our biochemical make-up. Our health depends on whether our bodies can protect themselves from this vast array of chemical assault while at the same time dealing with food that is increasingly lower in quality – soil mineral levels are at an all-time low.

In the US, the Environmental Protection Agency (EPA) reported that over 70,000 chemicals are commonly used in foods, pesticides and drugs. Some 99 per cent of these chemicals did not exist 100 years ago – our bodies and genetic pool have not had time to adapt to all these toxins.

We live in a culture where fast food and processed foods dominate our supermarket shelves and refrigerators. These so-called 'foods' have low nutritional value and are tampered with in order to imitate the real thing. Food writer Felicity Lawrence has found that most ready-made chicken sandwiches contain poultry that has been injected with starch, water and flavourings to disguise its low meat content.

About £11.2 billion is spent each year on chemical additives to change the colour, texture and shelf-life of our food. And while the food industry may defend its use of additives by saying that they are protecting us from food poisoning, these additives account for only 1 per cent of the amount used – 90 per cent are solely for cosmetic purposes.

Our bodies are further stressed by constantly trying to adjust to chemical toxins in the air we breathe and water we drink, as well as those released from our thoughts and unexpressed emotions; all of which makes it difficult for our bodies to function at optimum levels and eventually results in illnesses that affect our mind, body, or both.

It is hard to imagine a period in the history of our planet when it has been such a polluted place – on an individual level this pollution attacks our bodies with every breath we take. One billion pounds of lead and 600,000 tons of pesticides and fertilizers are dumped into the atmosphere each day. Non-organic food is sprayed with pesticides to kill insects, but these also affect humans over time – and so by definition are also degenerating and lowering our vitality.

Many of these chemicals impair our body's immune system, leaving it open to infections and viruses. For a growing number of the population, weakened and overstressed immune systems cause an overreaction leading to auto-immune disorders such as allergies – and meanwhile our defence systems attack our own normal healthy cells.

Chemicals used on the skin are also being questioned, as reports now suggest that commonly used preservatives in cosmetics, such as parabens, are linked to breast cancer. They mimic the behaviour of oestrogen and are well-known irritants to the skin and eyes. Sodium lauryl sulphate has been found to damage protein formation in the eye tissues of young animals as well as penetrating the tissues of the brain, liver and heart through the skin – yet it is widely used in shampoo.

It's surprising that with all this information freely available, cosmetics companies still pursue our bodies with 'nanotechnology' – biochemical product compounds with the ability to penetrate deep into the protective layers of the skin. These compounds are already being used in the manufacture of sunscreens, but the real aim of this technology is to exert more pharmaceutical influence on our bodies, in the sense that these products will not only change the appearance of our skin but lay a permanent imprint in our bodies. It's disturbing that in the US this technology arrived in department stores without first having undergone the usual clinical trials that could reveal possible side-effects.

Overwork and poor work surroundings compound these environmental factors, and have been blamed for a raft of stress-related illnesses. At present in the UK there are about 64,000 stress cases waiting to go through the courts. Government statistics reveal that 13 million working days a year are lost to stress-related illness in Britain, which adds up to £3.5 billion in lost revenue.

Self-inflicted Stress

Our drive to acquire material wealth in the hope of maintaining social status pushes many people to take on more than their physical and mental systems can cope with. Surveys constantly attribute the growth of stress to money and relationship problems, bereavement, moving home, serious illness or even having a baby (and its reverse, fertility problems). These factors also form the basis of a seething general level of anxiety and depression that occupies the minds of millions and fuels the massive anti-depressant drug industry.

Anxiety is different from stress in the sense that it comes from a lack of control over circumstances. Occasionally, this can produce solutions to problems, but usually it simply results in negative thinking and a defeatist attitude.

And yet, not all stress is negative – without some sense of drive and a good dose of adrenaline some things simply would never get done. We would lose interest and become demotivated. Life is and will be full of testing situations that should stimulate us to dig deeper and know ourselves, but it is how we *deal* with this stimulation that can cause trouble. Problems usually start when there is little opportunity to unwind from stress, and the battering of adrenaline and other stress hormones causes the body to attack itself, draining its vital systems and spiritual energy for life.

Unlike all bygone ages, life is still inherently stressful for many, even though obvious diseases and illness that previously ravaged generations, such as cholera, typhoid and all the poxes, are under control. We tend not to notice when our body is under this subtle but dynamic form of attack, and often let this pressure build up.

We spend so little time reflecting about the quality of our lives and the decisions we make that problems can get out of control – being stressed decreases our problem-solving abilities; stress chemicals and hormones impair and cloud our reasoning powers.

This cycle is vicious because by the time we realize we have a problem or are in trouble, we often feel too low to deal with it mentally. Life becomes a mist from which there is very little relief, and many people suffer in silence – that is, until the body forces a complete slow-down in the form of a health scare that helps us to reassess our lifestyle and health.

All too often we keep going for long periods of time in pressurized situations when our bodies are only designed to cope with short bursts of stress. And because too few of us seek effective ways to ease this pressure we constantly live with, most of us 'adapt' and allow our bodies to adjust to the stress. Unfortunately, only a small number of us have a superhuman capacity to deal with long-term stress.

What I'm trying to illustrate here is that there are potentially very many layers of pressure hitting our bodies at any given time, which accumulates to form stress. If we live in an emotional, physical and mental fast lane, then when obstacles arrive we'll have little time to put the brakes on – or our vision will become so blinkered that we will be unable to see how to alter our course positively.

Inflexibility and a lack of vision to welcome change are short-sighted and unrealistic – possessions and material things do not make us happy or last for ever, so always trying to hold onto them is likely to end in suffering. In truth, possessions and our relationships with them are in a constant process of change. By developing a wider view of life that nurtures more parts of ourselves, we learn to let go and accept that not every aspect of life is under our control.

Stress Makes Us Fatter

Our natural 'flight or fight' urge exists to help us either flee or do battle with potential enemies. Under stress our hearts start pounding, which increases blood pressure; blood is then diverted to the muscles, which slows down digestion, and breathing becomes shallower. We start to sweat to control over-heating, muscles tense up for action, and fats and sugars are fired into the blood to provide fuel. And finally the hormone cortisol is released from the adrenal glands – its job being to thicken the blood to help it clot at injury sites and to cool inflammation.

This effect is useful when the body is in a traumatic situation like starvation, bleeding or pain from surgery, but excessive and prolonged cortisol release disturbs our internal physical systems. One of the problems with excessive amounts of cortisol in the blood is that unlike growth hormone or testosterone, it breaks down muscle tissue – it is essentially helping us to become weaker and fatter.

In Chapter 4 I will talk about the necessity for weight-bearing exercise, as it helps to maintain a good metabolic rate and muscular strength, but when long-term stress is added to the equation of poor nutrition and no exercise, it becomes easier to understand how our lifestyle has contributed to an increasingly obese population.

An excessive amount of cortisol slows down our metabolic rate by converting proteins from muscle tissue into glucose to feed the body. This is necessary when the stomach is essentially placed 'out of order', as blood needs to be used by the muscles rather than the digestion. The less dense and inactive muscle tissue we have, the slower the metabolic rate and the fatter our body becomes.

In its initial stages, being stressed actually makes us more alert, but our bodies should not be in this condition for too long – it compromises normal bodily functions, leaving the body open to real foreign invaders like viruses. Daytime 'brain fog', high blood pressure, heart disease, ageing of the skin, allergies, insomnia and impaired immune function are just some of the effects of cortisol intoxication, while some of us may encounter feelings of complete exhaustion.

Clients (of mine) who are stressed tend to become very argumentative even when they are trying to do something positive about their health. They often become indiscriminate about their food intake at a time when mindfulness and positive food choices could help to reduce their stress levels. Some develop large, rounded and hard stomachs due to their body's inability to digest the food they rush to eat during long working days.

Undigested toxic waste simply sits in the body until medication to combat constipation relieves what could develop into a long-term colon problem. The inability to digest food tends to be one of the most common by-products of stress, because our bodies become locked into an adrenaline cycle. This stress and the adrenaline burn up large amounts of energy, increasing the body's demand for food while at the same time shutting down the digestive system.

As the body runs out of energy it will send out strong messages to refuel quickly, usually resulting in a sugar fix – simple carbohydrates like sugar do not require much stomach acid to digest. Many clients have spoken with me about their constant sugar cravings. But for many, eating this way results in weight gain due to the high volumes of insulin released into the body, which again slows down metabolism.

New research, however, disputes that the messages we receive from our body are for sugar per se. When under stress the body will initially demand more food because the hormones released speed up the heart rate, thus increasing the metabolism. But the craving for sugar is really a call for easily digestible food, which could be met with fruit, soup or with complex carbohydrates such as rice, sweet potatoes, cooked vegetables or oats. These foods provide the necessary energy required by the body, without destabilizing fluctuating blood sugar levels.

Although some people experience weight gain when stressed, for others, in more advanced stages of stress-related physiological changes, a great deal of weight loss can occur. The more highly stressed you are, the more probable it is that you will lose your appetite altogether. In a highly stressed body, blood supply to the stomach becomes so restricted that little stomach acid is produced – it is this amount of acid that stimulates hunger. Consequently, many people who suffer long-term stress can suffer equally from ulceration/inflammation of the colon and from malnutrition.

As a trainer, more often than not I encounter the type of person who has gained weight with stress and this has been partly due to impaired judgement about what they should eat and drink when experiencing stress. Their pattern tends to involve eating foods that are high in either fat or sugar or both, followed by a constant need for stimulants like caffeine or alcohol – eventually creating their very own fairground ride, rolling on uppers and downers, seeking comfort to get them through the day and evening.

However tempting it is to hit the bottle, this is unhelpful as alcohol on top of anxiety further aggravates the body's adrenaline response, disrupting both sleep patterns and blood sugar levels. Also, drinking on an empty stomach can weaken the muscle lining further because it keeps the top and bottom of the stomach taut, making it more prone to heartburn.

Likewise, starting the day with caffeine is not a good idea as it sets the heart racing and destabilizes the emotions, when in fact water and a nutritious breakfast would help to cool and calm the body properly to prepare for a challenging day. Sugary foods at the beginning of the day, such as honey-coated cereals or pastries, cause blood sugar levels to surge high then low, exacerbating mood swings, and have even been known to trigger panic attacks!

Coupled with the muscle-destroying effects of cortisol, stress makes a powerful fat-creating system supporting both the junk food and diet industries; not to mention the pharmaceutical companies who push their happiness and stress-release pills onto the nation in their millions.

In an ideal world, if you can recognize when you are in a stressful situation, whether long- or short-term, there are several immediate steps that can be taken to readdress and limit its effects on the body during the day.

1. Increase your water intake; eat vegetable soup, salads, nuts, seeds and oily fish to cool your body down.

2. Simplify your food intake: white meat, fish, fruit, vegetables and rice are easiest to digest.

3. Practise a deep-breathing technique first thing in the morning, in the middle of a stressful day or before you sleep at night. It really helps clear your head and relax your body.

4. To regulate your heart rate and help in the elimination of excessive amounts of stress hormones in the blood, do some form of light- or medium-intensity aerobic exercise morning or evening – this could even be a walk home at the end of the day.

5. Try to stretch out or have your body massaged to help release tightened muscles.

STRESS CONTROL: BREATHING AND MEDITATION

Stress not only causes our muscles to tighten involuntarily, but our breathing becomes more rapid and shallow – to ease this we need to use deep-breathing techniques that regulate our respiratory system and help it to return to its normal breathing rhythm. Stress shortens normal breathing patterns, which decreases the volume of oxygen supplied to the body. Less oxygen to the brain can result in the early death of brain cells and cause degenerative conditions like senility. To a lesser extent, this same lack of oxygen causes the digestive system to become sluggish and incapable of absorbing nutrients efficiently.

In such cases I have found light aerobic exercise to be beneficial, because when working out, greater and deeper volumes of oxygen are used, which regulate breathing.

If you are too stressed to start a regular exercise programme, you can use a deep-breathing technique for at least 20–30 minutes once a day to regulate your heart rate out of the stress zone. I have often advised stressed clients to go dancing, take long walks or simply sit in a dark room for the allotted time at the end or beginning of the day to practise breathing.

By deep breathing, I mean that air is taken into the lower abdomen so that it extends for a minimum of 10 seconds, and exhaled for the same length of time, making the stomach small. This is not an automatic reflex action but requires practice and concentration.

Here are four steps to deep-breathing practice:

1. Find a place that is calm, or a favourite place in your home.

2. Sit upright with your legs uncrossed, either on a chair or on the bed with your back fully supported and hands resting on your thighs.

3. Close your eyes and start by taking in breaths of 4 seconds and exhaling for 4 seconds until this occurs naturally, and concentrate on the counting. If thoughts about the day enter

your head, just focus your mind back onto the counting and breathing.

4. Repeat this process until you feel your body relax and can easily perform counts of 15 or more.

Deep breathing works particularly well when stretching or whenever you feel the need to clear your head – at work, just before you go to bed or as a 'time-out' in a challenging day.

Deep breathing is an excellent precursor to meditation – used together they are powerful stress-busters. The type of meditation I advocate is based on a mixture of breathing, visualization, colour therapy and positive affirmations. These require no mystical commitment but are based on Western self-awareness and mind-development practices. For me, meditation is invaluable 'me time' that eases my sometimes over-stimulated life – all of us need the peace to hear ourselves and get off the roller-coaster of life positively.

Until this point I have looked at the effects of stress on the body, but it is our minds that are the major producers of toxic and negative matter that causes the release of damaging stress hormones. The instruction to release cortisol into the body takes place in the brain as a direct result of the way we perceive problems and challenges.

Mental stress created by anxiety and negative thoughts goes on to produce negative reactions in the body. When anxious we tend to interpret even ordinary everyday situations as threatening – and this is usually rooted in fear and poor self-confidence. It is commonly shown that stressed adults have a constant stream of negative self-talk going on inside their heads that makes it difficult for them to perceive their situation as anything other than bad.

These issues could include work changes, body image, money problems or difficult emotional and family ties. Meditation reduces the primary source of stress, which is anxiety.

Ironically, it is precisely when stressed that we most need to slow down, but we find it difficult to actually sit down and reason out our problems, because the adrenaline flowing through our bodies creates the need to 'fight or flee'. It requires a certain amount of self-discipline to actually do the opposite.

High levels of stress hormones in our bodies lessen our response to demanding situations; we become slower and less efficient when compared with those with low stress levels. This also leaves us with no reserves for situations when they are really needed. In reality, stress often leads to substance abuse and a reliance on coffee, nicotine, alcohol or drugs to release strain, all of which offer only temporary respite.

If possible we should meditate daily, so that when confronted by anxiety and stress a partial cure is already in place, thus lessening the chance of potential cortisol and adrenaline release – it is preventative as well as healing.

Meditation creates time for the mind to rest by consciously trying to clear the clutter of everyday issues. This is not to say that you should try not to think; quite the reverse: you should attempt to think only of that which is positive and restful. Over time, practising meditation allows your body to heal as metabolism, heart rate, blood pressure and muscle tension all decrease. Your brain waves will actually shift from the fast beta waves that occur normally during the day to the slower alpha waves that dominate when we are truly at rest.

Research has shown that meditation significantly helps both athletes and those suffering from personality disorders that cause emotional insecurity and a lack of self-confidence. For instance, a study by the British Sports Council in 2000 looked at distance runners who had meditated for six months and compared them with a controlled group over the same period who had not.

Those who meditated were found to have reduced levels of fatigue in the form of less lactate, and lower lymphocyte levels (both of which diminish performance and affect the immune system) than those who did not. Hard training weakens the immune system; transcendental meditation was found to alleviate stress not only on the immune system but also on the way in which physical stress was experienced.

Other studies suggest that meditation is effective at dealing with stress hormones because, like exercise, it can reduce the production of and help clear cortisol from the brain. It also increases the production of 'happy hormones' such as serotonin. Higher serotonin levels increase an inner sense of security, decreasing the anxiety that causes many to feel that they cannot cope – remember, the less stressed you are, the more clear and precise your judgment will be.

There is no right or wrong way to meditate. It may be listening to music, while cleaning the house or doing what many of you might think of as the habit of 'day-dreaming'.

Three types of meditation are considered to be of therapeutic value:

1. Transcendental Meditation – founded by Yogi Maharishi Mahesh, uses repeated short words or phrases to clear the mind of extraneous thoughts to achieve a state of deep relaxation

2. Mindfulness Meditation – practised by Buddhists, asks the mind to focus attention non-judgementally on the present moment by pushing the breath on to other bodily sensations

3. Relaxation response – this is a physiological state brought about by several approaches including meditation and other relaxation exercises to counterbalance the body's normal response to stress.

You can start to practise meditation simply by following the steps I've listed below. It is important to clear your environment of any clutter and make sure that you feel comfortable; I like to light a scented candle, burn lavender incense or have some flowers around, as they lift my spirits after a hard day.

Many clients find it difficult to meditate at night due to tiredness, so practise in the morning. But make sure that you are fully awake whatever time you choose, as you need to be able to steer your mind down positive pathways. Although you should be relaxed, the aim is not to sleep during the session.

1. Find a place that is calm, or a favourite place in your home.

2. Sit upright with your legs uncrossed, either on a chair or on the bed with your back fully supported and hands resting on the thighs.

3. Close your eyes and start by taking in breaths of 4 seconds and breathing out for 4 seconds until this occurs naturally. Concentrate on the counting. If thoughts about the day enter your head, just focus your mind back onto the counting and breathing.

4. Repeat this process until you feel your body relax and you can easily perform counts of 15 or more.

5. Once your mind is clear and your body relaxed, continue the breathing style but not the counting.

6. Imagine a white light flowing down into your body from the sky, through the top of your head down to your toes.

7. Focus on this light for as long as possible, with the energy flowing out of your toes into the earth.

8. To combat stress, try to think of the deepest blue colour in front of your closed eyes. Allow the blue to move over your head and eventually over your whole body.

9. At this point, any affirmations that promote a sense of emotional and physical health can be repeated. Some examples you might like to use are: 'I have an abundance of wealth for all my needs;' 'My mood is calm and relaxed, my body is healthy and strong;' 'I have the clarity and courage to deal with all the challenges in my life.'

10. Finally, to end the session, imagine yourself emerging from a pool of clear blue water while still connected to the white light at the top of your head.

11. Take three deep breaths and open your eyes

This entire process can take anything from 30 minutes to an hour – the aim is to stay in that place of calm for as long as possible. Like most forms of training it needs to be practised regularly for the benefits to be felt, so start with a short time and then build up to as much as you need.

The effects of meditation are permanent because when used with positive affirmations to deal with fears and insecurity it actually heals the deep causes of stress rather than just the symptoms.

Although I have not gone into detail about the use of colour or aromatherapy here, there are several excellent books on the market, listed in the Bibliography. I have only given you an example of how colour and smell can be used in meditation to enhance the goal of relaxation; with practice you will be able to make up your own procedure to suit your individual needs. You must do what feels right for you and accept this information as a starting point.

STRETCHING

Given the effects of stress on the body, it is important to have techniques and practices in our lives that combat its damage every day. Prevention is better than cure – without an active relaxation programme we are more likely to become stressed. I have found two stress-busting techniques to be incredibly effective – stretching and meditation. Both help to normalize imbalances in our mind and body, while stretching specifically helps to correct postural problems which further strain our skeletons.

Tense, tight muscles perform poorly and affect the functioning of our vulnerable internal organs, which in turn causes the body to use excessive amounts of energy simply to move around. Flexible, healthy muscle tissue needs to be able to lengthen and contract with ease to supply our skeletons with a frame that supports movement – without soft tissue our bodies would be unable to move.

Like the other forms of exercise which will be discussed in Chapter 4, a structured stretching programme should be performed weekly as part of a basic body-maintenance and fitness strategy. Yet it is the most neglected part of most exercise routines because the outward benefits are less visible and, unlike weight training or aerobics, it does not necessarily produce an endorphin high or carry social kudos. You rarely hear someone say, 'Hey, you look really lengthened and stretched-out.' We tend to interpret well-balanced de-stressed bodies as having 'an elegant bearing' or belonging to a person who 'moves gracefully'.

We are at our most flexible between the ages of seven and 12, then during adolescence flexibility tends to level off and even starts to decline. After the age of 25 normal ageing tends to speed up, causing marked changes in our connective tissue, which eventually decrease our ability to stretch. With old age, collagen fibres thicken and the bonds within this structure strengthen, making it more resistant to all forms of movement, be they elongation or just everyday movements. And as dehydration in soft tissue structures also rises with age, this lack of water produces less lubrication and a poor flow of nutrients to these sites, which ultimately creates more fragile joints.

Stretching is key to keeping a constant supply of blood and nutrients to joints as it aids the flow of lubrication in the form of synovial fluid within the joint capsule. Stretching also helps to decrease the risk of injury during physical activity.

This is why it is so important to develop and maintain a movement programme as early as possible in our lives – the more mobile and flexible we are when young, the more likely we are to remain this way as we grow older. Inactivity promotes shortening within connective tissue and makes it less resilient and more dry, often resulting in poor muscular balance, which is essential for proper alignment. Given this state of affairs, we are then more likely to tear and damage our bodies as we age.

Although men can achieve great levels of flexibility if they train effectively from an early age, women tend to be more flexible. Men tend to have particularly poor flexibility around the pelvic girdle whereas women are super-flexible here – scientists generally agree that this is largely to accommodate child-bearing. The hormone *relaxin* softens and relaxes ligaments for a greater range of motion during pregnancy, so that there is space for the child in the pelvic region. Also, women are more flexible due to their active lifestyles and, when young, are more likely to take part in sports such as dance, gymnastics and ballet, all of which include some form of flexibility training.

Hang Loose – How Stretching Works

Flexibility training involves exercises that help us to maintain a full range of movement around our joints, which helps to neutralize the everyday wear and tear that may cause our bodies to shrink prematurely or inhibit us from reaching our peak physical potential.

To be flexible means that a joint can move freely through a pre-set, full and normal range of motion (ROM). Within each joint and for every activity there is an optimum ROM. For example, if I want to kick a ball across a football pitch, it would be essential that my knee and hip joints have full range of movement in order to produce the power for the ball to travel the distance with speed and height. Without this full range of joint movement, my performance would be compromised.

However, we are not all created equally – some people genetically have a greater or lesser level of joint mobility due to the quality of their connective tissue, the elasticity within the muscles or simply the level of mind–body co-ordination. With training, some of these factors can be modified to help balance muscles that are overused – not only during training sessions or sport but also as a result of poor posture – but not all.

To stretch we need to apply force to a limb to overcome resistance within the joint, which will eventually increase its range of movement. For some, this process can be difficult, not because of a lack of flexibility within the muscles but largely due to the connective tissue in and around the framework of the muscles, i.e. the tendons, ligaments, etc.

Connective tissue is made up of collagen fibres, which are a hard protein material that also has a high pliable strength, enough to support and protect soft tissue structure like muscles and internal organs. We can improve these fibres through training because connective tissue has two properties: it is elastic (in the sense that, if elongated, it can spring back to its original shape) and it is plastic (after tension is applied it remains in the newly elongated shape).

This is important to remember because so many of us believe that we're inflexible and that this cannot change, when in fact the reverse is closer to the truth. Like most exercises, the more you practise stretching, the greater the results and improvement in the body.

Adequate training should be designed to gain not only elastic but also plastic elongation, which is best achieved through static stretching – exerting a low force over a long duration: that is, 20 seconds or more.

Warming up is essential for successful stretching – it will help to minimize structural weakness and prevent permanent damaging elongation such as pulled hamstrings or torn ligaments. If you try to stretch without first warming up, you can expect to strain or tear the very tissue you're trying develop.

You can use both static and dynamic forms of stretching, but they'll only help your overall fitness if done in the appropriate environment and with adequate training. Dancers performing the splits – a move that shows the full ROM around the hip joint in a stationary position – use static stretches. Gymnasts performing high kicks or leaps use dynamic flexibility – these moves are dependent on resistance to motion at the joint and involve speed.

I agree with the fitness industry which now advocates that stretching *prior* to activity is not necessary – it should take place *after* a workout, for two reasons. First, when our body's core temperature increases and is at its highest point, muscle and connective tissues are less resistant, so produce maximum gains when stretched. Also, after exercise, muscles may have adapted to a shortening position and are tightened due to repetitive contraction. For instance, after running all match long, a professional footballer's hamstrings become very tight and are then prone to damage – they need to be stretched to remain flexible. Once muscles are warm, stretching the hamstrings brings the muscle back to its resting length and assists in the removal of unwanted waste products from the blood, like lactic acid, which can cause muscle soreness.

To prevent muscles tearing and tendons being pulled away from bones, our bodies have a sophisticated mechanism called *the stretch reflex*. This acts as a safety valve in muscle tissue, helping to prevent muscle tissue from tearing when excessive force is applied – it's a psycho-physiological process.

When a muscle fibre stretches, so does the adjacent muscle spindle. If the movement is extreme, the muscle spindle responds by sending a signal to the spinal cord, which returns an order to create a sudden protective muscular contraction.

The spindle ceases to fire as the muscle fibre contracts, thereby preventing tissue damage. An example of this reflex act is what happens if we fall asleep in an upright position. As our head relaxes and drops forward, the muscle spindle experiences a sudden stretch, sending a message to the cerebral muscle fibres, causing contraction and a sudden jerk to the upright position.

However, if the time and the force placed on the muscle become too strong, enough to risk rupture, contraction will stop. The muscle will relax as the Golgi tendon organ overrides messages given to the brain by the muscle spindle.

Stretching like this requires focus and knowledge of the stretching mechanism in order to recognize the messages being sent to the brain to achieve plastic elongation without damage. I've seen gym members bouncing on stretches as well as not remaining in a stretch long enough to allow the body to create either elastic or plastic development. Hence many think that they have tried stretching with little success, as they remain inflexible. It takes time, and in many ways yoga classes have facilitated the creation of a forum that allows ample scope for us to develop these stretches based on mental discipline.

YOGA

Yoga has been great at making us aware that we need to slow down in order for our bodies to recuperate from the pressures of everyday life. Like structured Western exercise it speeds up the use of oxygen in the body by using postures for stretching and deep-breathing techniques. The respiratory system expands its muscles down and out when air is drawn into the lungs, then pushes in and up during exhalation, allowing the lungs to expand to their full capacity.

This is not a reflex action but requires practice through concentration and relaxation. Also, yoga's stretching system gently speeds up the pace of the body and is very accessible – you can go to classes or exercise at home. But its arrival in the West has not been without its problems.

Yoga is a holistic system, directly applicable to the society in which it was created, and I for one don't believe that its precepts should be fragmented. What has developed in the West is a type of 'yogism' divorced from its spiritual base and dissipated into a mass of divergent forms, which often neglect the essential meditation component. True to form, many who practise these newer brands of yoga gain only partial growth and not its full benefits – there are more effective ways of changing the body or of losing weight.

I also question its recommendation for generalized dietary purification through vegetarianism, as often people do not have enough nutritional knowledge to eat balanced non-meat meals. Eating like this often ends up creating nutritional deficiencies and eating disorders, which can lead to serious health problems.

The information I've given on stretching is the minimum required for you to develop post-exercise or as a separate component of your weekly workout (more about this in Chapter 4). Yet few yoga teachers can explain or protect their students from over-elongation injuries, and may actually push students to attempt postures that are completely out of the range of their capabilities.

Yoga has helped to show that mind–body co-ordination is improved by stretching, as it makes our central nervous system more aware of the physical demands placed on it, helping muscles to work in a more synergistic fashion. This reduces muscle soreness and helps to realign soft tissue structures like tendons and ligaments which may have adapted poorly to the effects of gravity, causing bad postural habits.

Prior to the yoga explosion in the West, most stretching techniques were taught after aerobic/keep-fit classes or existed as pre-exercise warm-ups. Today the benefits of stretching are recognized as going far beyond just helping to return the body back to its pre-workout state; they also help to release stress built up by the body's own stress hormones which cause involuntary muscle contractions that then generate anxiety.

Stretching is integral to any relaxation or fitness system, and should be practised regularly.

POSTURE

I believe that the way our bodies move in everyday life affects our general level of stress and health. If we cannot perform simple tasks like walking or carrying the shopping comfortably, we are not heeding the signals of potential problems with our long-term health – our posture is often the signature of general health.

We often think of the upper part of the body as the base of good posture, but many major imbalances actually originate in the feet. Our feet are the foundation upon which all movement in our body rests, yet imbalance and defective mechanical function cause many adults to live in pain, unable to access a full vocabulary of physical expression. Poorly functioning feet result in all movement from the base of the body upwards to be flawed.

If feet over-pronate – that is, roll in towards the centre of the foot when moving – it is usually the result of the loss of the arch on the inside. This can cause pain through the ankle, knee, hip and lower back. It can also inflame the joint of the big toe to form what is commonly known as a bunion, and lead to unequal incorrect use of the muscles in the leg.

Pronation problems cause many of us to feel that we are not of the right make-up to experience exercise without pain. It's an extremely common problem, usually noticeable in adults whose foot arches have dropped with age. Often it will result in a gait where the knees knock or collapse towards each other. Wearing insoles tailor-made to create an arch, thus taking pressure off the inside of the foot prior to exercise, helps to heal pronation imbalance. It is absolutely necessary to have a foot assessment with a podiatrist to see whether your feet are in neutral alignment before you start an exercise programme. This will ensure that no further damage is caused to your feet and that your gait is secure for successful movement development.

In recent years elongation and strengthening techniques such as Pilates have caught on to the need for exercise that helps us to turn inwards and focus on our own body's structure as a whole – with an emphasis on the dynamics of posture and correct body alignment.

Pilates focuses on correcting postural imbalances and on how muscle supports the body to provide a balanced frame. Bad posture and poor spinal function compromise movement and inhibit the way internal organs can work to optimum levels.

For instance, if a person has rounded shoulders and a sunken chest, this will make it difficult for them to breathe deeply. The chest muscles are under-used while the back muscles are overused and constantly stretched. Opening the chest through a mixture of stretching and weight-bearing exercises helps the chest function correctly by holding the upper body upright, which in turn allows the back to support only those muscles on its side without strain.

For supporters of the Alexander Technique, good health is not merely seen as the absence of sickness or concern for the size of muscles and thinness of tissue, but valued at how well we bear our body-weight.

As a technique I have found it fascinating that, with practice, simple movements can help to alleviate a multitude of problems. Matthias Alexander, through his own inability to speak after an accident, discovered that by changing the position of his head, then body, pulling it upwards, the negative effects of gravity could be counteracted. It was these negative results that went some way to produce a rounding of the spine and shoulder muscles, which in turn caused the head to be pulled backwards and down. According to Sarah Barker in her book on the Alexander Technique, 'This is the first destructive habit, the first of a whole series that will follow, if it goes unchallenged.' What's more, from this moment on all movement becomes an adaptation to this structural defect. Simple actions like walking, running, lifting shopping, bending to pick up a shoe, getting dressed and even brushing our teeth are then performed in a poor way as a result.

Incorrectly aligned everyday tasks become harmful as they compress discs in the spine and cause our bodies to waste energy. Repeated hundreds of times a day, within a very few years this interferes with the smooth running of our muscular–nervous systems and vital organs. And for some of us this results in round-the-clock tension in some muscles, high blood pressure and chronic joint pains.

Healing occurs when the neck is repeatedly prevented from contracting unnecessarily, which requires using our conscious mind to change our subconscious (often learned) muscle patterns. This approach involves bringing forward and acknowledging subconscious sensations to the conscious mind, so that with every act we consciously move our head upwards, with the body following it.

For example, when you are seated, your back and shoulders should not be rounded with a collapsed abdomen and neck over-extended forward and down. Instead, the head and back need to be upright with the neck relaxed, shoulders back, chest up, so that your abdominal muscles can have space under the lungs to reside comfortably, supporting the spine.

The whole aim of a balanced frame is to have a body that functions with maximum ease and co-ordination, so that the only effort used is that which is absolutely necessary. This is Alexander's definition of 'good use', while 'bad use' equates to employing the body in a haphazard way: one part compensating at random, usually inefficiently, for the movement of another in order to maintain balance and stability.

Critics of Alexander's work call his principles 'idealistic' because it is difficult to talk about the 'idea' of posture – which in the Technique relates to a stationary point and does not truly reflect the action of real life. Life itself consists of movement, and nothing is stationary. They believe that, in its purest form, the word can be applied only to the rare occasions when one may adopt a stance before coming into a room or when one is poised at the head of the stairs. Once you start to move down the stairs you are caught up in movement and the way you usually hold your body will reassert itself immediately.

While there is an element of truth in these criticisms of the Alexander Technique, we can retrain ourselves to employ 'good movement' consciously, and to maintain this throughout our daily lives. For example, most sportspeople have good posture due to the exercises they perform daily so that their bodies are balanced both in and out of their sport – there is no transition.

Ideally, the erect body should provide enough room for internal organs to be massaged by our breathing. If the body is slumped, unnecessary pressure is placed on our organs, which slows circulation. Likewise with the spine, if the vertebrae are stacked unevenly, the pressure of the body being supported by them will not be evenly shared and some parts of the spinal cord itself will experience undue pressure. This may result in nerves being pinched, which causes the malfunctioning of the parts of your body serviced by them – for example, you may experience 'pins and needles' or numbness in your legs.

We have to become more aware of the way we use our bodies for movement in our everyday lives, and back this up with solid exercise programmes that support the continuous activity of daily life. Our bodies should be lengthened and balanced in the performance of common actions like walking, sitting, lifting objects or climbing stairs.

If we try to push the body erect forcibly, we can cause some muscles to overstretch while dramatically shortening others. This is why the Alexander Technique involves the slow physical *and* mental process of repeating basic actions that help to relax previously strained and stressed muscles.

The Alexander Technique works wonders on soft tissue but it does not really address movement problems or unexplained pain due to structural defects in the hard matter of the joints – it is not an appropriate practice for those with structural problems.

Many people believe that their movement quality is bad simply because that is the way they were born, but usually when you look back at your 'physical history', you may have suffered injuries that have caused structural damage – joints or bone may have been reset in a way that prohibits movement. Your body has adapted to the new, less effective or efficient mode of action that has created poor-quality movement.

All soft-tissue manipulation has its limits if the internal structure of your body is weak – healing needs to start internally so as not to compound already established problems. No act of mental will or gentle movement can enable a person to stand tall or get rid of back pain if movement is stopped or prohibited by live connective tissue. Full and painless movement cannot be expected from the neck, for example, if the vertebrae are out of place – chiropractors use X-ray machines to get a clear view of the discs within the spine.

Accurate and precise diagnosis of defective joint tissues is so important – it's so easy to waste a lot of time, money and energy on ineffective soft-tissue techniques. Hard tissue or fascia changes can be helped through techniques used to manipulate the connective tissue and not the muscles, like those employed by chiropractors – who believe that the source of many muscular aches and pains actually develops from our 'second brain', the nervous system and spine.

While they agree with Alexander that excessive pressure on the spinal column causes stress and prevents effective movement of the body and its internal organs, chiropractors move the debate forward by stating that this is only the superficial stage of damage. They believe that pressure on the spine also causes delicate nerves to become pinched and inflamed.

Discs in the spinal column can and do move completely out of position, which over years causes the growth of collagen fibres over the entire joint capsule. To try to re-learn how to perform a movement that involves such a spinal joint would take a very long time. Chiropractors can locate the precise distressed or damaged disc, break the newly acquired collagen fibres and then place the disc and joint back into its original position so that the spine can function correctly. After this has been set and fully healed, the soft tissue of muscle can then be effectively re-trained to correct use.

It's not a painful process but you may require several treatments, because if a joint or disc has been fused for years due to poor alignment, it will not shift easily. Only by moving these joints repeatedly can we ensure that they will eventually stay put. This stage is then the right time to use soft-tissue techniques like Alexander's, Pilates or the gym – being active accelerates healing as controlled actions re-train and stabilize the joints. Being active can actually help with the early detection of imperfect joint action; with the right treatment these joints need not cause discomfort.

I believe we can maintain a balanced frame through various types of exercise. No one system holds 'all the truths' – *you* need to find the right technique to heal *your* body. I am both a soft- and hard-tissue practitioner because exercise heals and influences the joints, ligaments and muscles, while structured stretches support and lengthen the body.

Exercise helps you to maintain good movement in your everyday life, which reduces stress in your body daily – this assists you in keeping excellent posture. The creation of a balanced frame is no easy feat and requires a constant level of awareness – what you are thinking as well as how you are moving plays its role. Flexibility training and meditation are not only essential for our physical health but also vital for keeping our heads clear. Stress must be managed in positive ways so that challenges in life, be they physical or mental, do not become part and parcel of your life.

Chapter 3
Eating to Live

Feelings run high on the subject of food, and we live in an age that has seen unparalleled abundance in the choice and sheer volume of what we can eat.

This abundance is partly a direct result of our emphasis over the past couple of centuries on the advancement of human life, so that for the first time in history most of us in the West do not have to worry about where our next meal is coming from. Ironically, however, as we experience the bounty of nature's stores, nutrition-related illness grows and on the other side of the planet people are dying of starvation.

At the same time our culture remains confused about what we should eat, and state revenues suffer the burden of enormous healthcare bills for ever-increasing levels of preventable illness.

We are torn between eating for pleasure and eating simply to live – a choice made more difficult because of the steady barrage of advertising. A whole industry exists that shows us on television, in magazines and in books about the luxurious foods we could be eating – at home, at work or on holiday.

I want to shed some light on this confusion by looking at some major food issues and show you how to find a balance, so that you feel confident to eat in a way that will not compromise your health. Equally, with so much food readily available, one of the most challenging aspects of everyday life is how to prevent over-eating shortening your lifespan through obesity, high blood pressure, heart disease, arthritis, diabetes or cancer, rising levels of which are now prevalent in our culture.

TOO FAT OR TOO THIN?

Notions of balance and moderation, and attempts to eat what our body needs, appear to be out of control. I believe this to be symbolic of us being out of touch with ourselves. We're given contradictory messages about the true condition of public health. The press is littered with stories about anorexia and other eating disorders, but in reality the reverse is true for the majority of us – our bodies are carrying too much fat.

Children as young as six have been treated for eating disorders, but victims of eating disorders are usually women in their teens who are generally thought of as highly intelligent and high-achieving. The Eating Disorders Association suggests that there are 1.2 million sufferers in the UK. Over 90 per cent of people suffering from eating disorders are women, but the figures are steadily increasing for both women and men, to more than 7,000 per year.

Another, more publicized, influence on anorexia figures has been said to be media images of thin women – a generation ago a model weighed 8 per cent less than the average woman; now she weighs 23 per cent less. But it's not only fashion models whom women want to emulate: in today's culture, actresses, singers, dancers and many entertainers are all either digitally airbrushed down to childlike proportions, or choose to live on extremely low-calorie diets which compromise their health, just so they can maintain a palatable media image.

As long as these public figures continue to be revered for the way they look, some vulnerable women will feel pressure to emulate the illusion of thin as beautiful. Some 10–20 per cent of anorexics will die by suicide or create permanent damage to their kidneys, liver or heart through under-nourishment. A girl of 18 may lose 20 per cent of her bone density, effectively becoming as fragile as a 60-year-old.

Treated early, 75–90 per cent of women can recover from anorexia – a third within five years – but the remainder may only make partial recovery and many will be ill for 20 years or more.

If a woman survives an early brush with anorexia she may still join the three in every 100 women who are bulimic – a cycle of alternatively starving and bingeing that usually affects women in their twenties and thirties and is thought to be caused by traumatic childhood experiences. In 1994, 45 per cent of bulimic sufferers came from a background of being badly looked after by parents. Bulimia causes damage to the teeth (mottled by acid from the digestive juices), salivary glands and throat. Frequent vomiting can upset body fluid and electrolyte levels, leading to heart failure, kidney damage or epilepsy – death is usually the result in 10–20 per cent of cases.

Eating disorders compromise future health because instead of the body growing in preparation for later life, it is denied many essential nutrients, leading to the rise of other ailments like osteoporosis. One in three women and one in 12 men now suffer from a lack of minerals such as calcium, magnesium and zinc, exacerbated by sedentary living. In 1997 in the UK there were 60,000 broken hips, 50,000 broken wrists and 40,000 spinal fractures – all more common where mineral levels are low.

More women die indirectly as a result of osteoporosis than from cancer of the uterus, ovaries and cervix combined. Bone-wasting illness is rising by 10 per cent a year, and about 50 per cent of schoolgirls who have tried to diet and missed their period for just six months have increased their risk of the illness, as bone degeneration interferes with normal hormonal production.

Throughout my career I have encountered numerous cases of distorted body image in women – it is a recurring issue. While some women do not understand that the images they see are not real, others have unrealistic ideas about how they should look and so do not trust themselves to eat properly. They struggle to make eating nutritious food their number-one priority because they feel invisible if they do not conform to fashionable images, when in truth they need to stop feeding those external images and feed themselves properly instead.

Often I'll hear stories of a golden age when they were 'thin, lithe and could eat anything' – they appear to relish thoughts of possessing that type of body again. But, once again, this thinking about the true nature of their bodies is flawed and misguided. Like nature, all states of matter must and do change; the body at 20 years of age cannot and will not be the same as at 40. It will be different but it's still absolutely achievable, with care and maintenance, to have the best possible body you can have at any given age.

I feel there is little to gain from trying to recreate the past, and everything to live for by moving towards the future with a realistic, attainable vision of our bodies, based on the quality of material available in the here and now.

Going on starvation diets to lose weight fast produces more problems than they're worth, and will eventually undermine your long-term weight-loss efforts as it will slow down the rate at which calories are used by your body. Starvation diets contribute to the breakdown of lean muscle tissue, the very tissue that speeds up your metabolic rate, and they are very difficult to maintain for any length of time – which in turn promotes yo-yo dieting. Numerous studies have shown that initial weight lost usually returns more quickly once normal eating is resumed. The heavier you are, the more calories you need to maintain your size. A lighter person will need less food to remain at the same weight.

So, to lose weight, a heavier person needs to consume about 500 fewer calories a day for their body *at its initial weight.* Then, when they have lost some weight, they need to reduce their intake again, or increase their exercise output to allow for their smaller size. The volume of food a nine-stone person needs cannot satisfy a 12-stone person of similar height and physique – the greater the surface area, the greater the heat loss that occurs through the skin, which increases metabolic rate. On a practical level this means that heavier people have higher metabolic rates and need to eat more food than smaller people, as they have a greater surface area to maintain.

Apart from your metabolic rate, the other defining factor that influences the speed at which calories are used is the volume of energy expenditure – exercise – you take. If you eat and drink less food than you need to live on for energy, then your body has to draw on its own energy stores to survive. Ideally, this energy will come from your fat stores.

We forget that fat is only a type of fuel; if it is used or burned, it no longer exists. A healthy weight-loss programme should help to change poor dietary patterns by allowing the body to use up fat stores efficiently rather than lean muscle tissue or glycogen (a type of sugar in the blood).

Oddly enough, for many of my clients their weight problems are not due to overeating but to some of the habits mentioned above, so I have actually had to *persuade* them to eat. Many studies have shown that the act of eating speeds up the rate at which calories are burned in the body, due to what is called in scientific terms 'the thermic effect of feeding'. Digestion, absorption, breakdown and storage of food all require energy; not eating slows down the entire body's metabolic rate.

By eating beyond our body's needs and expending too little energy, our nation has become overweight, and this, coupled with its associated ailments, are the greatest problems facing the health service.

In Britain, obesity is increasing at an alarming rate. Some 45 per cent of men and 33 per cent of women are overweight, while 17 per cent of men and 20 per cent of women are clinically obese. Likewise, in the US, according to Professor Philip James, 61 per cent of the population is at least 30 lb overweight, with 21 per cent certified as clinically obese. This rate has more than doubled in the past 18 years. Millions of children's lives are at risk through soaring levels of Type II diabetes, and in 2002

Britain saw the first cases of Type II diabetes triggered by obesity in teenagers.

We no longer have the luxury of eating solely for pleasure, but must instead start to understand food as energy input. Yes, taking pleasure in food is part of our social heritage, but our health is our responsibility. Pleasure cannot be the only variable – if you have social events in a week that will be high-calorie, then you need to balance this with some exercise to help offset some of that gain.

Life was not always so for Britons; in 1954 the average size-12 woman weighed 8 stone 7 lb, compared with 9 stone 3 lb today. On average, in terms of energy intake we are eating 25 per cent less than we did when wartime rationing was still in force in the 1940s. This illustrates that the majority of food we eat must be high in fat and sugar, which, in tandem with a gross lack of exercise, has caused our health to deteriorate.

It is this fine balance between exercise and what we put into our bodies that generally determines our state of health. Finding equilibrium is an individual process. No two bodies are exactly alike and, therefore, do not use the fuel of food in exactly the same way.

What you eat influences the quality of the information your mind produces – some of us have become so disconnected we can no longer rely on our minds to relay reliable messages about even simple things such as whether we are hungry or not. So, increasingly, we eat foods that are not good for us – high-sugar, high-fat foods that result in feelings of guilt, heaviness and stagnancy. For others, food has become a type of therapy that comforts us, an anaesthetic for the pain and floods of emotions raging through our bodies.

The anxiety and pressure of low self-esteem, work, stress or relationship crises are all too often drowned in bottles of wine, drugs or binges of so called 'gourmet' fast foods. Once the body has been subjected to repetitious cycles of nutritional abuse, it is hardly surprising that its internal wiring becomes jammed, unable to communicate clearly with the mind and divorced from being able to discern which foods are needed for health.

Without the necessary education on how to care for our bodies, many suffer in silence with negative eating and lifestyle patterns until illness forces investigation into the body's shutdown.

ALCOHOL

It is not just food that is influencing our present health problems. Britain currently faces a torrent of alcohol-related illness to the tune of £1.7 billion – the human cost has been a seven-fold increase in deaths from liver disease among women aged 35 to 44. According to Alcohol Concern, over 3 million people in the UK are dependent on alcohol.

Although the media have focused on the resulting poor social behaviour, I think we also need to look at the fact that a lot of alcohol manufacturers have increased the strength of their products. They have increasingly marketed their goods to a vulnerable younger audience (who have little knowledge of the long-term damage alcohol can cause their bodies) – sugary alcoholic drinks nicknamed 'alcopops'.

The level of alcohol in wine has risen to 12 or 13 per cent, as opposed to the 9 per cent that was traditionally standard. Raising the strength of alcohol in drinks makes it more difficult for us to regulate how many units we are drinking, which is one reason why bingeing has become more prevalent. Health guidelines state that women should only drink two to three units of alcohol a day, but today this equates to just one and a half glasses of 12 per cent wine or two single measures of spirits – few stay within this target in an evening and the norm is more likely to be double this at least. Of women who drink, the proportion who drink above the safe limit is over 70 per cent.

Binges are helping to create the increase in overweight women because, after fat, which has a calorific value of 9 calories per gram, alcohol is the next most fattening substance we consume, with 7 calories per gram. Protein and carbohydrates have only 4 calories per gram. The calories of alcohol are also 'empty' in the sense that they provide energy but nothing else – no vitamins or minerals and no fibre. These empty calories can themselves lead to artificial feelings of hunger as they produce a rapid rise in blood-sugar levels followed by an equally sudden drop, which then reinforces a cycle of poor nutrition, as it creates cravings for fatty foods.

Wine, in particular, helps to stimulate appetite by encouraging gastric secretion. So not only are women making themselves feel artificially hungry, they are also consuming poor-quality calories while bingeing on alcohol and destabilizing their blood-sugar levels. This taxes the pancreas, making it produce more insulin to cope with the high levels of sugar in the body. Insulin, coupled with eating more fatty foods, makes for more fat storage on internal organs and in the body.

On the whole, men are better equipped to deal with alcohol in their bodies than women are, and have to abuse their bodies for a long time before they actually develop health problems. Physiologically this is because women's bodies tend to absorb more alcohol than men of similar build. Women have less effective stomach enzyme activity, which in turn makes them more prone to liver disease than men.

Men's bodies are also better at breaking down fatty acids that accumulate around the liver than are women's. The inability to think straight after taking alcohol is significantly greater in women than men, which is why television footage of adults vomiting in the streets or, indeed, collapsed on pavements, tends to be of women.

At a metabolic level, women find it more difficult to eliminate toxins from their bodies, because the rate at which they use calories is slower than for men. Compared to men, women's bodies are smaller, carry less fat-free mass, and tend to be colder, all of which make for a base metabolic rate that is on average five to ten per cent lower than men's. Women also tend to suffer from hormonal problems that can again slow down the base metabolic rate and produce mood swings and artificial cravings for foods they would not consume if their hormone levels were normal.

Additionally, excessive drinking decreases vitamin absorption; drinkers are likely to eat fewer fruits and vegetables, resulting in poor nutrition or even malnutrition. For the body to break down alcohol it must generate free radicals – negative oxygen molecules – which in turn leads to premature ageing. If all of this were not bad enough, heavy drinking interferes with our ability to reproduce; as much as 40 per cent of male sub-fertility has been blamed on an alcohol intake of just five units a day. Not drinking improves sperm counts and sex drive in both groups within three months.

To my mind, binge drinkers are either consciously or subconsciously opting out of responsibility for their bodies and need to look at the underlying issues that cause such self-harm. They know it is not beneficial to their health, but if asked why they continue to take part in such a pastime, many will answer that they simply love to have fun that way.

I question whether such a health compromise can lead to happiness. Even a superficial investigation into many of these people's lives reveals that they are, in fact, unbalanced: trying to run away from feelings of pain or addicted to the euphoria in a bottle while failing to confront life issues they wish simply to anaesthetize away. Perhaps they are suffering from personal loss, work, financial or emotional trauma, or spiritual crisis of some sort which, for one reason or another, they feel they cannot deal with in a more positive way.

Our bodies were not built to deal with such large amounts of toxins, especially as environmental ones like pollution and everyday carcinogens are challenge enough. If alcohol intake to such high levels was positive for the system, then we would be a healthy nation. Instead, most of us have lived enough to have suffered the massive drawback of a 'hangover from hell' coupled with days of depression and just feeling weak, as the body tries to recover from the physical battering. Binges may have resulted for some in an increased risk of liver psoriasis, high blood pressure and unwanted pregnancy as well as cancers of the mouth, breast and colon.

Recent controversial research investigating the link between rising breast-cancer rates and alcohol has produced some interesting results. High levels of oestrogen in the body are thought to influence many breast cancers because while the liver is occupied with processing alcohol it cannot process oestrogen properly, which is thought to promote the growth of tumours.

Enlightened choices are possible, even in the most pressured social setting, without having to do away with either sugar or alcohol altogether. Awareness of the processes taking place in your body can help you make informed selections to limit the damage and stress put on the liver, brain, pancreas and blood. Listed below are a few tips on how to enjoy alcohol without the damage.

- Eat before you drink. This slows down the effect of alcohol on your blood-sugar levels – if going out for dinner, have a small snack first as this will help you to drink less while waiting for your food.

- Try not to drink high-sugar cocktails – these are not only high in calories but will cause your blood-sugar levels to skyrocket and then plummet, further weakening your will power against junk foods later on. Good-quality wines, pure spirits with fruit juice or low-calorie mixers are better choices.

- Keep your body hydrated by drinking water with alcohol – this will help to prevent the general inflammation that causes hangover symptoms like headache, dry tongue, bloated stomach and brain fog.

- High-fat foods on top of high-sugar drinks are a recipe for high body fat, so steer clear of junk foods like crisps, salted nuts, kebabs, chips, curries and ice cream if you want to keep your waistline!

- Low-fat foods like fruit, yoghurt, unsalted nuts, oatcakes, chicken, eggs and vegetables all help to balance your blood-sugar levels – if you have a couple of these ready at home after a night out you'll feel less hungry the morning after. A big fry-up isn't the only hangover cure.

- If you've had a heavy night drinking, try to rest the following day to allow your body time to process and recover from toxin overload. Focus on cooling your body – eat plenty of green vegetables, lean white proteins and salads as well as peppermint, camomile, lavender or milk thistle tea.

What I am trying to highlight here is not abstinence, but rather the idea that we all have a choice about how we want to treat our bodies. We need to act as if we understand that substances like alcohol can damage us if used inappropriately – alcohol is not a food but a drug. Excessive intake stresses you both physically and mentally – if your body is occupied with defending itself against toxins it will have little strength to deal with real diseases and infections.

EATING PATTERNS

Only in recent years have we begun to take on board what are good foods for the body and what constitutes a positive eating pattern.

More often than not, my clients will have been eating poor-quality foods grabbed at the end of a busy day with very little in between apart from diuretics and stimulants like coffee or cola. We still fail to link up our poor dietary habits with constant tiredness, stress and perhaps the inability to meet the physical or mental challenges of everyday life. With so much food on offer, it's still surprising how little variety we have in our diets. Many find themselves stuck in a rut of no breakfast, constant sandwiches and alcoholic dinners. Or we feel too mentally 'fried' at the end of a day to think about food. Instead we try to get away with relying on parts or pieces of the food chain to remain healthy.

All foods provide energy to power every activity of cell activity and growth in the body. This energy is measured in kilocalories (kcal). The total number of calories in a food depends on how much protein, fat and carbohydrate it contains. Every gram of fat contains nine calories; a gram of protein or carbohydrate has four calories. Hence a diet too rich in fats encourages weight gain as it will have more calories that one based on a mixture of all three food groups.

Today nutritionists would advocate average energy input of around 2,000 kcal for women and 2,500 for men, but in my experience these figures are generally too high. Something in the region of 1,500 calories a day for women and 2,000 for men will maintain most people's normal healthy weight. Although we are mentally fast, physically our lifestyles are slow. And these guidelines will be further affected by individual genetics, lifestyle, height, weight, age and muscle–fat ratio factors.

The equation for weight loss is not complicated: *if the energy consumed in food is less than the energy used in physical activity, body weight will decrease.* Food consumed cannot disappear; if unused it will be turned into fat and stored in the body. To lose weight, less food must be eaten than is required for the body to live, or it must be used up in activity. To maintain your body weight, you simply eat the same as the energy use.

The above equation tends to work for the majority of the population, but there are people who will not respond or who are exceptions to these rules. This group includes people with hormonal imbalances, which includes the growing number of women suffering from the stress-related illness called PCOS (Polycystic Ovary Syndrome), those with under- or overactive thyroid glands and people with high levels of fat-free mass (i.e. muscle), or those on certain types of medication.

It is thought that eating small meals often actually helps to keep our metabolic rate high so that we don't feel as if we're being deprived of food. It is now widely accepted that this way of eating, coupled with a suitable exercise programme, discourages fat production. Unfortunately, I think this way of eating produces a false sense of security in many and actually encourages overeating. I think the point of such research was to show that large meals or starving the body slows down the metabolic rate – but eating three meals a day of the calories the body needs will not make it put on weight. These studies simply advise us of an eating pattern that could help us to use our calories more efficiently throughout the day.

THE MENSTRUAL CYCLE

A woman's monthly menstrual cycle, hormonal imbalances and emotional problems can make it even more difficult to keep to a healthy eating plan. However, it is possible for us to improve and manage hormonal shifts by stabilizing blood-sugar levels with phyto-oestrogens and balanced aerobic exercise.

I find it slightly disconcerting that some manufacturers play on women's vulnerability with myths that we need to eat large quantities of chocolate to help us through our 'time of the month'. Without a second thought, manufacturers push their high-sugar and high-fat merchandise, then look away from the obesity, self-hatred and bad health they have helped to create.

Like most, I enjoy chocolate but this treat should be eaten in moderation, and I always opt for a pure, organic kind. It should not be used as a main food source, especially at a time when your body requires wholesome nutrition that will stabilize and nurture it during the stressful part of the month.

Our menstrual cycle allows us to rotate naturally the number of calories consumed each month without altering our overall calorie intake, which helps to stimulate high metabolism.

Before menstruation, most women have a reduced appetite and eat quite sparingly, while post-ovulation decreasing levels of the hormone oestrogen cause an increase in appetite. Eating high-quality, low-glycaemic carbohydrates, portions of lean protein and several helpings of vegetables per meal helps to balance blood-sugar levels without accumulating extra body fat.

We can ruin a great month's worth of workouts with repeated chocolate or other junk food binges around the time of our period, resulting in a lot of frustration and depression.

Bingeing is often a sign of deeper emotional turmoil that becomes particularly active at this time in the month. Worry, financial anxiety or relationship issues tend to loom large under the influence of these hormonal changes; it is necessary to face these issues before eating problems can be tackled effectively.

Excessive heat or cold can also speed up the rate at which calories are used by the body, while ageing slows down calorie expenditure by about two to five per cent per decade after 40 in both women and men with sedentary lifestyles.

A HEALTHY PLAN

The easiest way to help maintain an ideal weight is to make structured exercise an essential part of your everyday life and couple this with a healthy eating plan. Few of us have the time or energy to work out exactly how many calories we need to eat to lose weight and, to be honest, minor fluctuations don't really count – it is more important to structure the big picture of your lifestyle, then you can allow yourself to break the rules occasionally.

First you need to get a handle on whether you are eating too much or eating healthily in relationship to your lifestyle by going through the figures. Figures provide a guide, revealing in black and white just where over- or under-eating has been taking place, and help show obvious nutrient imbalances. Once a new pattern has been established and you see the results, number-crunching becomes unnecessary and you'll be able to hear true messages from your body of hunger and satiety.

Hunger and the feelings of being full are like red and green traffic signals that sometimes receive interference from our external environment and emotions. Stress, happiness and temperature all influence what and how much food we eat.

When we are anxious, the temptation is to eat fatty comfort foods to tame the bubbling sensation that's created in the stomach. Some researchers believe that eating in this way produces 'stress fat' on some overweight people. There are few people who have not reached for the chocolate, chips, crisps, ice cream, alcohol or indeed the large variety of junk foods to calm frazzled nerves – but poor eating patterns only compound mental stress.

There are two issues that need to be tackled to prevent this type of excess calorie intake. First, you have to recognize and, if possible, deal with, the environmental or emotional issues that are creating your stomach disturbance. Then you need to decide whether or not food will solve this issue. It may sound complicated, but you'll soon get used to your mind and body becoming engaged in honest dialogue that allows you to deal with matters that upset you.

For example, whenever I had to do some sort of public speaking, or teach large groups of people, I got really bad nerves. I suffered a bad bubbling in my stomach to the extent that it would eventually turn into a pain in the pit of the right side of my stomach.

I knew I couldn't be hungry because I'd just eaten, so I decided to investigate what it was about these situations that made my body anxious. I found that I had a fear of being not good enough and of being judged as mediocre, even though consciously I did not believe this. In my subconscious mind these thoughts had been floating around and would finally centre in my stomach when I least needed to deal with them. Even though I had no evidence to promote the negative thoughts that lived in my head, and in fact was always pleasantly surprised when the speaking went very well, I could not get rid of the bubbling.

Further consideration revealed that what was taking place was a form of stage fright and I decided to tackle it in various ways. First, I decided to confront my issues by re-training my mind not to produce such negative thoughts that would, in turn, upset my body. I achieved this through meditation, breathing techniques and positive visualization, and made sure I was always totally prepared for the sessions. Then I decided to ensure my stomach had enough alkaline foods in it before giving a speech. Alkaline foods absorb stomach acid and ensure a constant blood-sugar level. Eating lean protein with green vegetables or salad with brown rice, followed by fruit, secured stable energy levels. Although coffee or tea was often offered to me beforehand, I learned not to drink any form of stimulant, as these only added to the surges of adrenaline already in my body.

Consequently, upset stomachs and performance doubts are a thing of the past, to the extent that I now look forward to and have grown to love public interaction. This is one example of how emotions, environment and food work together and have to be considered as a whole. My response to performance was a psychological pattern I recognized but broke in order to move forward – it was never a food problem even though it was activated in my stomach.

Overeating must be looked at in a similar way, addressing your situation and mental patterns. Once these are redressed, distinguishing the signals of when to eat or not will become easier, and eventually poor food choices will no longer be a substitute or cover-up for underlying emotional issues.

A food diary is a very informative and useful tool for anyone who feels they need to eat more healthily, because the process of recording all you eat immediately creates a shift in awareness. Recording what we eat changes our eating patterns in a positive way. Information is key if we are to make our food work for us.

As regards 'balance', I use the word advisedly because what's a balanced nutritious meal for one person may be highly disruptive to another. It is a myth that all foods are nutritious for all humans. What is one man's food is definitely another man's poison, so you need to take the time to find out what foods are best for *you*. Famed proponents of this position are Dr Peter D'Adamo and Catherine Whitney in *Eat Right for Your Type*. They emphasize the importance of having knowledge about blood type and the role that it plays in creating food intolerances and allergies.

To maintain health we need to have a balanced diet that utilizes a wide variety of nutrients from different parts of the food chain, as they rely on each other synergistically to provide energy for the body's needs. Food can be seen in terms of macronutrients (carbohydrates, proteins and fats which provide energy for daily activities and contain calories) and micronutrients (water, vitamins, minerals and fibre, which carry little or no calorific value but play a major part in energy-producing chemical reactions in the body). The two types are interdependent: neither can fully produce the true extent of their value without the other.

I cannot stress this point strongly enough. There are so many diets on the market that advocate the withdrawal of one or many nutrients to achieve weight loss. These are unhealthy and, except in cases of particular medical conditions, they should be viewed with suspicion. Such diets are unsustainable and usually constructed around ideas of starvation or detoxification.

FOOD GROUPS AND HOW THEY WORK

Protein

Protein is crucial for the growth and repair of cells in the body. It is responsible for healthy bones, red blood cells and skin, and is an essential component of muscle. It serves as the structural basis of all enzymes and hormones that control basic functions in the body. You need to eat foods like meat, fish, eggs, milk, tofu, pulses, nuts and seeds every day – but don't rely on one type; mix both animal and vegetable sources to remain healthy.

With nearly half the calories of fat (only four in comparison to nine per gram), protein increases the metabolic rate when eaten and tends to satisfy hunger more readily as it takes the body longer to break down. But eating too much will not be used in the body to build more muscle tissue; instead, it will be converted and stored as fat.

Too much protein promotes dehydration, stressing the kidneys and liver and increasing calcium loss. For these reasons I view high-protein diets with suspicion, and nutritionists generally view them as unhealthy. These diets are not helpful for the majority of us who in fact need to follow long-term healthy-eating plans that are sustainable and do not risk our health.

On average we need only one gram of protein per kilo of weight, so if you weigh 65 kg, then 65 grams of protein can be eaten per day from a mixture of animal and vegetable sources. Animal protein should be eaten in its most unprocessed and organic form because the nutritional value of a piece of chicken will always be higher than in processed or ready-made varieties filled with preservatives, hormones and antibiotics.

Carbohydrates

Carbs include starches such as potatoes, bread, some peas, beans and pasta, and sugars found naturally in fruits (fructose), refined as granulated sugar and in milk as lactose. They have the same calorific value as protein (four kcal per gram) but affect our blood-sugar levels, which, in turn, positively or negatively influence our overall metabolic rate.

All carbohydrate is changed into glucose in the blood and this raises the blood-sugar levels to provide energy; any excess is stored in the liver and muscles as glycogen. When these stores are full, the excess is converted to and stored as fat. Our bodies must turn dietary carbohydrates into glycogen, as dietary glycogen does not exist outside our bodies.

Many overweight issues usually start here, because eating only slightly too much generally, together with a lack in exercise, will make us fatter over time – in past times our bodies would have stored excess fuel for lean days when there would have been a lack of food.

The body prefers to use blood and liver glycogen for energy rather than fat, because this type of sugar is made from linking glucose molecules rather than fat molecules together – which is an easier feeding process.

The modern sedentary lifestyle provides little need for the body to reconvert fat to sugar for energy unless we exercise (see Chapter 4), so we need to make wise choices regarding starchy foods. I use the word 'wise' because research has shown that it is not only the volume of carbohydrates we eat that contributes to balancing blood-sugar levels but also whether they release their sugar around the body quickly or slowly.

Nutritionists such as Dr Antony Leeds rank carbohydrates according to their immediate effect on the blood-sugar level. This ranking, called the glycaemic index (GI) of foods, can help determine how quickly they break down in digestion – fast being a high GI, while slow absorption has a low GI ranking as it releases glucose gradually into the bloodstream. Keeping a moderate and constant blood-sugar level is desirable because when levels are too high, the pancreas secretes more insulin – a process that slows down the body's metabolic rate, thus increasing weight.

Carbohydrate stimulates the secretion of insulin more than any other type of food. A carbohydrate slowly absorbed into the body stops the pancreas from working so hard and produces less insulin. And the gradual rise and fall in blood sugar helps to delay and manage hunger pangs. High levels of blood insulin followed by a sudden drop triggers the release of serotonin (the feel-good hormone in the brain) to let us know that we are full. But eating foods that create high insulin levels reduces our ability to experience this cut-off point, so we're left feeling rarely satisfied by our food.

While the glycaemic index for food has been helpful in highlighting that all carbohydrates do not have the same influence on the body, as well as the great role insulin plays in the creation of fat, it can be misleading.

The GI does not take into account the average portion size. You would have to eat a large portion of carrots (75 grams), for instance, for it to have a high sugar-rush effect on blood-sugar levels. Most of us would only normally consume between 20 and 30 grams in a meal. Meanwhile a dessertspoon of maple syrup – a pure sugar – would produce an almost instant 'high', but has the same GI ranking as the 75g of carrots.

Also, a striking problem is that fats and high-fibre foods eaten with carbohydrates slow down the absorption of sugars and help to create satiety. A mango has a GI of 55 (medium to high ranking) but is full of micronutrients like beta-carotene, vitamins and soluble fibre. When the fibre has been extracted from the equation it has just 19 grams of absorbable carbohydrate, which would lower its GI ranking. Mango juice or puree, on the other hand, would have a higher ranking than the raw fruit. The processing of food affects its GI ranking, often invalidating many of the values listed in tables, to the extent that their practical value is limited for users who need to know more than the net carbohydrate value of foods.

These anomalies have forced nutritionists to look back to the complete load of carbohydrate in relation to portion size, meal combinations and whether the food eaten is raw or processed – now termed the glycaemic load (GL). This is a useful dietary tool as it helps us to create balanced meals by looking at the whole of what we eat rather than its parts.

The most high-profile protagonist in the carbohydrate debate is Dr Robert C Atkins, with his books *New Diet Revolution* and *Atkins for Life*. His controversial diet and nutritional recommendations go a lot further than controlling the types of carbohydrates eaten, and involve cutting carbohydrates to five grams a day for the first two weeks of the diet! This allows the body to go into a process of ketosis, produced by the consumption of high volumes of protein. The process of ketosis allows the body to burn fat for fuel and produces rapid weight loss. After the initial stage, low glycaemic carbs are reintroduced back into the diet to help maintain weight loss.

This way of eating has helped many people to change their eating habits and successfully lose weight. It is an extreme measure for those who really have tried to change their eating patterns and failed because they are so addicted to sugars/starches. This is the real issue Atkins confronts: he effectively 'cold-turkeys' people off the high-starch foods many are so addicted to.

Before Atkins the public had little awareness about the effects of starchy foods on their bodies. While most dietary therapists focus on emotional issues that lead to over-eating, research now backs up the idea that certain foods are physically addictive.

Atkins has been criticized for recklessly promoting increased consumption of deadly saturated fats and overloading the kidneys by greater protein intake, but to date there has been little medical research to back up these charges. Nevertheless, there are now more moderate versions of his principles littering the diet market.

Although I do not agree with this diet, Atkins did prove that it was not fat that was making us overweight but rather too much insulin in our blood due to carbohydrate. He showed that the food pyramid advocated since the 1960s, which advised a high-carbohydrate diet rich in grains, potatoes and cereals, should be defunct. He also took stimulants like caffeine and alcohol out of the diet and promoted the use of low-starch vegetables and salads so that you feel less hungry. The appetite becomes re-trained and is stabilized to the extent that you actually eat less food, too.

The most important insight to come out of both Atkins's and Dr Leeds's work is that at this stage in our society's development there is a need to reduce the volume and type of carbohydrate being consumed to control our weight and remain healthy – many nutritionists now follow their lead, even if they have criticized their work.

The naturopath Dr Robert D'Adamo in *Eat Right for Your Type* offers a final but nonetheless vital piece of the carbohydrate puzzle. With his theory of blood types he adds to the debate concerning the effect of different foods in the body. He argues that we all have a different response to similar foods by the nature of our blood group (O, A, B or AB). This response has been genetically predetermined, and if foods carry unfriendly lectins (a type of protein that is carried on all foods) into the blood, which glue together in the stomach or internal organs, they can cause illness.

Foods help to create modern ailments like irritable bowel syndrome (IBS), migraines and asthma, which, over time, build into food intolerances. For instance, the carbohydrate wheat has a powerful protein in it called gluten, which is also a harmful lectin to those with blood type O. When consumed it blocks up their stomach and is believed to cause constipation and irritable bowel as well as contributing to weight gain due to the body's inability to digest it properly.

I suffered from all these complaints until I stopped following the advice of numerous doctors and nutritionists constantly advising me to eat more fibre and whole grains (Os also have little tolerance to nearly all grains) and found a naturopath. It's important to note that this system does not involve the expulsion of the food group carbohydrate, only to eating the types that do not produce this reaction, like the large variety of root vegetables, fruit, pulses and beans. Ailments like IBS, stomach cramps, eczema and asthma disappeared once I found out which foods carried unfavourable lectins for *me*, but these are different for different blood types. I have found the same to be true for many women and clients who have reached a plateau in their weight loss, which turns out to be not fat-related but toxin-based.

Dr D'Adamo is not advocating cutting out or even reducing carbs in the diet but, rather, each of us finding out which foods truly nourish the body because they are easy to digest. Foods that cause high lectin activity stress the body and contribute to ill health – heavy reliance on wheat or dairy produce can create this response.

His nutritional system has been successful because at its heart it is supporting eating unprocessed, balanced meals which, coupled with exercise, heal the body and promote health. At no point does he advise the dismissal of any food group out of everyday eating but clearly states, after years of research, that as humans we cannot all eat and break down the same foods.

Differences in our genetic code make it impossible for us to do this safely – the person of African descent will not have built up the same food tolerances as, say, someone of Asian descent. I find D'Adamo's work fascinating because it challenges an almost imperialist attitude that we should be able to consume all that the globe has to offer without question.

Again, his nutritional system has been highly criticized for being based on unverifiable anthropological theories, although these criticisms have largely fallen on deaf ears as thousands of people have found it helpful in curing many medical ailments without the need for drug intervention.

I do not think that to maintain a healthy diet it is necessary to go on Atkins, Blood type or GI programmes – all provide partial solutions to the very complex health problems that exist in our age.

Recently there has been a lot of research on the effects of high levels of sugar on the mind, and this has helped scientists to understand why low-carbohydrate diets are so popular. According to the New York University School of Medicine, too much sugar in the blood is causing the brain to shrink. The part of the brain called the hippocampus, which deals with memory, shrinks under the influence of high blood sugar and performs worse in short-term memory tests than brains with normal blood sugar. High blood sugar, unregulated by insulin, actually starves the brain of fuel so that instead of feeding it, it ends up shrinking.

We can all relate to this. It is what usually happens on Christmas Day or after big Sunday lunches, where it is usual to indulge in a carb feast – meals end in little conversation but everyone complaining of wanting to sleep as we can barely string a sentence together! Below I've summarized a few points to remember when eating carbs:

- Try to eat low-GI carbs like porridge, pitta bread and low-sugar wholegrain cereal for breakfast or lunch when your body needs energy most.

- Add nuts, seeds and protein to all your meals to stabilize blood-sugar levels.

- Control your portion size – your palm is about the right size of starch you should be eating in a meal.

- Remember that fruits, beans, peas, pulses, vegetables and some nuts are all high in carbohydrate but have added fibre which will provide a slow release of energy in your body – don't become reliant on grains or sugar.

Fats

Until fairly recently we believed fats to be a menace to healthy eating and the cause of increased weight, but fats play an important role in maintaining health and in fact help to reduce weight. There is little evidence that a high-fat diet actually causes an increase in bad fats in the blood, and today debate centres on which are the so-called 'good' or 'bad' fats.

However, eating a high-fat diet will contribute to making you over-fat as it is a high-energy nutrient – fats have an energy value of nine calories per gram, over double that of protein or carbohydrate. Nutritionists recommend that intake of fats should be approximately 33 per cent of our daily intake of food. If your daily dietary intake is about 1,500 calories, then about 330 calories can come from fat, which is roughly 33 grams (you simply divide the number of calories by nine).

Good fat intake is essential to the body for hormone production, cell-wall structural development, aiding the digestion of certain vitamins and minerals and providing protection for internal organs. Our blood cholesterol levels (the amount of fat in the blood) can be measured to identify the level of risk to heart disease – the type of fats we eat, our individual genetic type or how active we are, affects this. If blood cholesterol levels are too high, it can be a sign that fat is being deposited around the arteries, which in turn can lead to the circulation of blood being interrupted (heart disease) or stopped (stroke, heart attack).

In the 1970s it was popular for nutritionists to recommend low-fat diets high in carbohydrate; the result has been that today we are fatter than ever before. These calculations were off the mark because vital information about the nature of carbohydrates in our body was not widely developed. So, combined with our sedentary lifestyle – the explosion of office work and the evolution of car use – the result is that we've got fatter.

Ironically, on both sides of the Atlantic our diets are still deficient in positive fats like the essential fatty acids (EFAs) Omega 3 and Omega 6. Because our bodies cannot produce these nutrients it is essential that we eat them from seeds and unsalted nuts, green leafy vegetables and cold-water oily fish such as salmon, herring, sardines and tuna. They normalize blood pressure, help keep depression and hyperactivity at bay, as well as heart disease and cancer – they also reduce clots in the bloodstream. 'Good fats' like the EFAs are considered to be those that do not raise cholesterol levels and aid its removal from the blood. These come in two types, monounsaturated (found in avocados and olive and rapeseed oils) and polyunsaturated (nuts, seeds and sunflower oils).

Several studies show that long-term restriction of these good fats is quite ineffective for weight loss – eating high-fat natural foods like nuts can help reduce blood cholesterol and assist in satisfying the appetite, thus reducing overall food intake and stimulating the metabolism.

It is not eating fat that makes you fatter, but the *type* and *amount* of fat that are important – a view shared by several eminent cardiologists. As far as I'm concerned, it does not make sense to overload your body with large amounts of saturated fats found in animal-based products like butter, cream, fatty meats, cheese, processed meats such as sausages, cakes, biscuits and savoury snacks. Most clinical research shows that while it is valid for everyone to keep their intake of saturated fat low for good health (and that those with a family history of raised cholesterol should be particularly vigilant), there is little or no relationship between the intake of dietary fat and body weight.

However, when it comes to bad fats, trans-fatty acids (or trans-fats), made when hydrogen is added to oils to give them a solid form – such as in margarines – are top of the list. These fats, which are found in many processed foods like cakes and biscuits as well as numerous processed foods, do not melt at room temperature. While trans-fats were initially thought to have no worse effect on blood cholesterol levels than saturated fats, several studies have shown that they lower levels of HDLs (high-density lipoproteins, which protect the body from heart disease), are highly poisonous and even carcinogenic.

Specialists even believe that there is a link between trans-fats and brain damage, as they block the junctions of nerve cells, interrupting signals throughout the brain and body. A diet high in Omega 3 fatty acids performs the opposite function by aiding message transmission. Scientists believe that trans-fats have contributed to the increase in dyslexia and hyperactivity in children.

It is ironic that in the midst of the current obesity crisis the American food industry still allows the development and sale of so-called 'fake fats'. Olestra, a trans-fat approved for use in so-called low-fat snack foods, is synthetic and cannot be digested by the body. It passes through the body's digestive system, taking with it the fat-soluble vitamins A, D, E and K as well as a group of nutrients called carotenoids that play a vital role in the prevention of cancer and heart disease. Anal leakage, stomach cramps and restricted vitamin absorption are accepted as a price worth paying by an overweight population as long as it is supporting a cash-hungry low-fat diet industry.

These products continue to be made even though the US Food Standards Agency recently announced that these fats could be worse than saturated ones. The next time you pick up a health bar, margarine or ice cream sold from a van, remember the potential damage that will result.

Fake fats and low-fat processed foods tend to encourage our appetite for junk foods instead of for healthier snacks like fruit and vegetables. So many naturally low-fat foods, which are nutrient-rich, are readily available in convenient packaging, like pulses, beans and whole grains. Yet we still choose to eat low-fat ready-made meals, believing them to be the healthy option, when in fact they tend to be low in fibre, high in carbohydrate, too high in salt and containing only low-grade protein.

The overriding message about fats is that they are not necessarily the culprit behind overweight or illness; evidence for this presently points the blame at too much starch and too little exercise. But this is by no means a licence for you to indulge regularly in meals with high saturated-fat content – they are not healthy and contribute to metabolic stress and weight increase. Because they are high in calories, the emphasis should be on eating small amounts of the beneficial types of fats. We should seek to rid our diets of trans- and fake fats that compromise our health, and instead eat more unprocessed foods and take advantage of the great natural diversity of foods on offer to promote health.

Vitamins and Minerals

Vitamins and minerals form a major part of the micronutrient group; they are found in fruit, vegetables, nuts and seeds. They carry few to no calories but most literature argues that modern diets tend to be deficient in them. Some 15 vitamins and eight to ten amino acids are essential to normal body function. They are synergistic and without them no chemical reactions in the body would function correctly. They cannot be made or used by our bodies in their natural state, but are formed in minute quantities in all organic food, or can be obtained from dietary supplements.

Although severe deficiencies are rare in countries like the US and Britain, poor intakes of a number of these nutrients are recognized in 20 per cent of women of child-bearing age. The main debate around these nutrients centres on whether or not we need to use supplements, and many commentators would say the jury is still out. I believe the evidence suggests otherwise – supplements are a necessary aid to preserving health and restoring its balance.

The government recommends that the average person should eat five to seven portions a day of fresh fruit and vegetables, plus starches and protein to have a balanced, nutrient-rich diet. But many studies have proved that this is nowhere near the reality for most of us, who are regularly overdosing on junk foods with little variety in our everyday diet. Also, a healthy diet does not necessarily mean that the body is absorbing adequate levels of vitamins and minerals.

Stress, digestive problems, medication or recreational drugs can impair the body's ability to absorb food's goodness. Similarly, anti-nutrients (foods that provide little or short-term energy) like alcohol, caffeine and saturated fats not only add negative calorie intake but also deprive our bodies of the capacity to assimilate calcium, iron, magnesium and selenium – all of which are required for us to absorb other vitamins.

In addition to these problems we still have to consider the quality of the food on offer. We now live in an age where food can appear to be fresh and healthy when in fact it can be the most toxic product we could put into our bodies. The quality and value of non-organic fruit and vegetables have been depleted by the wide use of pesticides and cheap fertilizers; research has shown that the soil plants grow in no longer contains the minerals for plants to take up. In 1949, for example, 100g of spinach had 158mg of iron; now it has 1mg. Also, the same spinach may have been flown from Spain to Britain – 958 miles – and lost much of its goodness along the way. Spinach can lose up to 90 per cent of its vitamin C in the 24 hours after harvest.

Pesticides and the irradiation of foods offer the appearance of life, when in fact this food has little to no life-giving energy. Such food is just a shell of what it used to be and of very little use to the body. Friends of the Earth found that a typical lettuce will have been sprayed 11 times while it was growing; potatoes had 12 applications and a Cox apple up to 16 in season. Such food can be stored longer, and looks good, yet most of its vitamins will have been lost.

Non-organic animal products are full of hormones and antibiotics which have little positive effect on the consumer. Thousands of tonnes of such chicken is eaten in Britain, flown in from Thailand, a trip of 6,643 miles. Yet at the same time, Britain exports thousands of tonnes of this same product to the rest of the world!

The emergence of farmers' markets selling organic fresh foods has been only a partial answer to questionable supermarket foods, because the produce is so expensive. So it is still fairly difficult, given the pressures of life, to achieve the right balance of micronutrients. One would need to be a good mathematician and dietician to work out the daily volume of food needed, and then find time to prepare and cook it all! It is far easier to take a tablet with food – it may be not be the ideal solution, but it's practical.

We already know that eating too much food without adequate exercise helps us become overweight, so eating more food to fulfil mineral quotas would be simply encouraging people to get fatter. According to Dr A Walker, taking a supplement can help solve this problem. Neither do we need high doses; recent research has shown that, generally, the RDA (Recommended Dietary Allowances) dosages of vitamins and minerals are effective in helping to maintain health.

If a patient has an ailment or illness, therapeutic vitamin prescription is necessary, but serious harm can be done by high self-dosing. Research at Leicester University suggests that a daily vitamin C dose of just 500mg raises levels of a substance that may cause DNA damage, and possibly provoke the risk of cancers and diseases such as rheumatoid arthritis. For Sarah Schenker, a nutrition scientist at the British Nutrition Foundation:

> It seems that there is a kind of u-shaped progression here,
> where not enough of a nutrient heightens potential health risks.
> The RDA is good and lowers the risk of problems, but taking
> mega doses actually raises the risk of problems.[1]

For me, supplements are not a luxury but a necessity for both mental and physical health. We have little time, energy or inclination to find out how fresh food is, beyond it being organic and that it satisfies our urge to eat. If the food industry refuses to supply food in an acceptable condition, we have no choice but to attempt to make up the deficit as we see fit, without causing harm.

Again, micronutrients illustrate the need for us to eat real food as opposed to poor-quality junk or processed products. Real food, eaten in moderation, nurtures, heals and restores the body to a point of equilibrium – for optimum health, no part of the food chain can be omitted.

Water and Salt

Water is one of the most undervalued and underused micronutrients. On average we spend the best part of our day dehydrated through taking diuretics like tea, coffee, alcohol or drugs, or eating too much protein. While our bodies can survive up to 50 days without eating, we can live but a few days without water. National Water Information research shows that nearly nine out of ten of us do not drink enough.

Some 45–70 per cent of total body weight is water, and women hold less than men, owing to their higher fat levels. Many of the body's fluids are made up of water, which acts as a transport system, taking ingredients to critical organs, and taking by-products such as toxins and waste out of the body. Our key fluid, blood, moves oxygen and nutrients around the body. Bodily fluids act as a lubricant for joints and eyes, help the act of swallowing and serve as a cushion for the nervous system. They also serve to regulate body temperature – sweat is a cooling mechanism.

Yet with all this activity constantly taking place, we often act as if our bodies are a water reservoir, whereas the opposite is true. There is continual water-loss – and if the body is dry, normal processes cannot take place. Hence constipation, dry-skin conditions, brain fog, tiredness, loss of appetite, dry mouth, heat intolerance and muscle ache are all too common.

How much water is required is dependent on your individual metabolism and environment, but the general recommendations are in the region of one-and-a-half to two litres of pure water a day, which is then regulated by the kidneys – more is needed if you drink a lot of alcohol and/or coffee.

The thirst mechanism tells us if our fluids are running low, and is an emergency response to dehydration, so water should be drunk regularly to prevent this response – most of us, though, tend to do the reverse. We interpret our thirst message as that of hunger, which is why I advise clients to drink before they eat to find out if they really are hungry – most find that the water stops the cravings and clears the head until they are really ready to eat.

Salt, or rather sodium chloride, also increases thirst, but at the same time causes the body to hold on to excess water and raises blood pressure, which in turn ups the chances of strokes. Most of the salt we eat comes from – yes, you've guessed it – processed foods like crisps, canned soups, meat products, breakfast cereals, bread and savoury snacks. A daily intake of just three to six grams of salt is recommended by health professionals.

TOP TIPS FOR HEALTHY EATING

1. Try to drink one-and-a-half to two litres of water a day, starting with at least half a litre in the morning *before* you drink any tea or coffee.

2. Remember that breakfast is the most important meal of the day. It should consist of protein, carbohydrate and good fats like linseed, walnut or pumpkin-seed oil. Skipping breakfast destabilizes blood-sugar levels, causing overeating later in the day.

3. Eat four small meals a day as opposed to one or two large, heavy meals. This speeds up your metabolic rate and supplies the body with a constant source of energy throughout the day.

4. Try to cook as many meals as possible yourself, as restaurant food is usually full of saturated fats, salt and a lot of sugar. The same goes for processed foods and ready-made meals; eat as few of these as possible. They're full of trans-fat and salt.

5. Get into the habit of checking food labels. Choose not only low-fat foods but also those with few additives, pesticides, antibiotics and preservatives.

6. Eat good fats more often, like those found in olive, linseed or walnut oil, herring, salmon, mackerel, sardines, nuts and seeds.

These clear bad fats from the arteries and cool inflammation in the body.

7. And yes, do eat a bit more protein. Two pieces a day of lean organic meat, fish, poultry or soya products feed your muscles, speed up your metabolism and create a greater feeling of satiety (fullness).

8. Eat fresh vegetables and fruits every day, as these low-glycaemic foods will nourish you and help stabilize blood-sugar levels. However, make sure you also take a simple, inexpensive multivitamin supplement daily.

9. Drink alcohol in moderation, even at social events, as it can increase the damage to an already overworked liver.

10. Exercise – it increases the nutritional value you get from the food you eat.

Chapter 4
Exercise for Heart and Soul

It is widely agreed that exercise will make you fit and enhance your body's ability to cope with stress and heal itself naturally. Confusion arises, however, about *what kind* of exercise is best. For example, back in the 1980s it was widely reported that we should perform aerobic exercise for 20 minutes, three times a week. My experience as a fitness instructor, however, has taught me that this regime would have very little impact on a body that requires major weight loss or needs to be de-stressed. Usually I train clients for double this time, but keep the intensity of the sessions the same. In this way, I've found that they all lose weight even if their diets are not perfect.

Thirty minutes of aerobic exercise five times a week is now the normal suggestion (American Council of Exercise). Again, I would argue that this is incorrect. You need to warm up for 10 minutes *before* aerobic exercise, so the workout would be 40 minutes in total. This, together with the results of all my findings, I've put together for you in this chapter.

A BODY IN BALANCE

Exercise acts as a balancing tool between what we eat and how we think – it affects both our bodies and our minds. For most of us this mind–body connection has been compromised, so we need exercise in our everyday lives to increase our sense of wellbeing and health.

In past times we did not have as many labour-saving devices as we have today, so our physical lives were very hard. The Industrial Revolution created machines and technology that not only reduced the need to toil the land, but also brought much work into automated factories, as well as mechanizing the work performed in the home and in offices. We became free to concentrate on material advancement.

Our body's evolution, however, has not developed as quickly, and today we still require a high level of movement to remain healthy – without exercise we would have to employ very strict dietary control to maintain a steady, healthy weight. The most efficient way to maintain health is through a combination of exercise and healthy eating.

Without the need to perform numerous labour-intensive tasks or having to travel great distances on foot, our physical energy output is low. Striving for improved living conditions has led to a lifestyle that is totally unchallenging physically and that contributes to the high levels of obesity and weight-related illnesses common today.

Nor is the situation helped by our general lack of a spiritual or religious philosophy that engages our bodies with movement as part of an everyday discipline. Our secular society provides no means by which we can regard our body and its need for movement as an inherent part of life. Both exercise and structured-movement classes are promoted in our culture as separate from, and not rooted in, any form of spiritual discourse, whereas in the East spiritual practice is usually married to a highly developed movement programme, particularly for those practising yoga.

In China, the practice of *tai chi* (great energy), originally developed in the 12th century by a Taoist priest, made its way out of the monasteries so that, by 1949, China's government promoted its practice as a preventative health regime now used by millions of Chinese daily.

Tai chi seeks to increase the flow of what is known as *chi*, or vital energy, around the body as well as to promote relaxation and meditation. Through its practice as part of the religion of Taoism, people become in tune with their own 'path' or 'way' through moderation, humility and integrity – attributes unlikely to appear high up on the educational curriculum of the average Brit.

Similarly, the Hindu religion has the physical practice of yoga, created as far back as the 3rd century BC. For its advocates there is no separation of mind and body, just a single organic whole. Both affect each other through our conscious will; hence it is emotional tension that often results in physical illness. Practitioners aim to gain a more relaxed response to emotional tension to aid wellbeing in order to discover the optimum potential that exists inside everyone. It is a mental and physical discipline that demands that the individual look inwards, away from the outside world, for knowledge of the self, while at the same time seeking connection with the universal spirit, or *prana*.

As with tai chi, yoga exercises or *asanas* are based on observations of animal life and are non-competitive (our sports, by comparison, are based on the ability to win – which means that someone also has to be the loser), with a strong emphasis on active relaxation/meditation that clears the mind of worldly stress. Hatha yoga outlines a system of healthy eating habits, high standards of personal hygiene, physical postures, breathing techniques and meditation to achieve pure consciousness.

Both Chinese and Ayurvedic medicine attempt to heal the body's energy centres via pressure points in a holistic way. We in the West did not look seriously at these principles until the second half of the 20th century, when they experienced a rather explosive growth. Now many Westerners practise these disciplines, hoping to achieve physical improvement without having to change spiritually.

Like The Star of Wealth, progress within these practices will be only partial if we do not change from the inside out – sustainable self-discovery can only be achieved if you apply yourself to all levels. Also, I believe that adopting Eastern philosophy and practice produces only limited results because they are culturally specific – tailor-made for the societies for which they were created.

Most of the inhabitants of these societies still have a fairly labour-intensive existence, hence their bodies require more rest from the strains of everyday life – it is this that makes yoga, for instance, beneficial for them.

In Britain we suffer from the opposite problem: stress and illness are increasingly caused by *mental* strain, a lack of the right type of physical movement and a poor diet. For me the benefit of yoga or tai chi can only be partial because, taken on their own, they do not offer enough respiratory exercise for our Western bodies. If there is one part of Eastern physical and spiritual practice that could be of substantial benefit to us, it is the practice of meditation, but this is the very part that is most often rejected and ill-maintained. The Star of Wealth, through its promotion of Western exercise practice, offers a proven movement system that will heal your body and balance your mental and emotional spheres.

MIND WORKOUT

Much has been written about the physical benefits of exercise, especially in connection with weight control and illness prevention, but there has been little emphasis on one of its primary benefits – *exercise is essential to optimum mental health*. For this fact alone it should become a crucial element of everyday life, rather than viewed as exceptional.

While some research has focused on how we feel during a workout, its after-effects and the role this plays in relation to stress release, others have looked at the quality of brain/cognitive power enhanced by working out. These studies are important because they suggest that being unhappy or forgetful, having a poor attention span or being thought of as not particularly intelligent are all related to a lack of movement. Over the years I've noticed that people who exercise regularly are generally happier, more confident and better able to cope with stress than those who do not. The whole experience of exercise itself produces a feeling of clarity and relaxation which I have found difficult to replicate in any other sphere of life.

Scientists have long theorized about endorphins in the brain creating euphoric sensations that are addictive, but I believe that the effects of exercise on the brain are a little more complex than this.

It's no coincidence that our culture's obesity problem is coupled with high levels of recreational drug/alcohol use and anti-depressant dependency. It is an indication that millions of people are finding it difficult to cope with modern life and are unhappy – not knowing why they feel so uneasy within their own skin and dissatisfied with life. They appear to need to cut off the feelings they experience in their bodies through substance abuse in order to tolerate life itself.

We spend millions trying to keep people mentally well, in addition to the billions spent on physical health problems caused by lack of exercise. A quarter of all drugs prescribed on the NHS are anti-depressants. Between 1990 and 1995, this figure rose by 116 per cent for the monoamine oxidize inhibitors (an enzyme that breaks down adrenaline and noradrenaline in the blood) and by 732 per cent for newer anti-depressants like Prozac (selective serotonin re-uptake inhibitors). According to the mental health charity Mind, 300 out of every 1,000 people experience mental health problems, and in 1999 ten per cent of children were diagnosed with some form of mental disorder.

On average in England there are 5,000 suicides a year, the biggest risk group being men between the ages of 25 and 35. In 1999 this represented a great change, as previously it was men over 65 years of age who were at the highest risk. It is interesting that instead of such wealthy times bringing us happiness, we have large numbers suffering the reverse. The second most common cause of death in men under 35 is suicide, and this trend appears to be on the rise.

In an attempt to address mental-health problems, the government recently introduced an initiative that advised GPs to cut back on prescription-drug therapy for depression. Doctors now advise exercise sessions, non-drug treatments and therapies. And yet there was no clear press campaign for their u-turn in policy. Yes, it would be nice to think they simply wanted to cut the NHS bill, but it is now apparent that more physiological knowledge about our bodies actually supported these initiatives.

National surveys carried out by Mind reveal that many people with mental health problems use exercise and physical activity to lift their mood and reduce stress, thus relieving the symptoms of depression. Moreover, exercise is already being used by millions as a preventative measure against mental illness. Yet little information has been given to the general public as to why this should be the case.

Scientists only recently discovered the physiological reason why exercise affects the mind positively. For many years it had been widely accepted that exercise was nature's anti-depressant, but now scientists have identified the actual chemical in the brain that produces this effect, and how it works in our bodies.

Nottingham University published research in the *British Journal of Sports Medicine* showing that the naturally produced chemical phenylethylamine was found to be low in the biological fluids of depressed patients. This chemical changes into phenylacetic acid, which tested low in depressed patients before exercise, but levels increased on average by 77 per cent after exercise.[1] Ironically, phenylacetic acid has a similar chemical structure to that of amphetamines, and is believed to be part of a 'runner's high' and of the chemical chain linked to natural endorphin activity in the brain.

Equally important is the fact that this acid can cross from the blood to the brain, something that endorphins cannot do, which indicates that it is more likely to be used in the body with ease. We need structured exercise programmes to elevate the heart rate beyond activities like walking, gardening, etc., because to produce the beneficial highs we need to exercise at a moderate to high intensity.

If further investigation proves the biological deficiency of phenylethylamine to be widespread, then the ramifications of this study and others like it are great. First, it would allow for thousands of those now classified as mentally ill to be re-categorized as physically ill. And while this already occurs for patients who are mentally ill due to dopamine imbalances, exercise could help to reduce the NHS's medication costs – which simply sedate the problem rather than offer any cure.

The government could then use the money saved to initiate an extensive educational programme to inform the public about the essential role movement plays in maintaining mental health. If people who use recreational drugs to stimulate dopamine and amphetamine responses knew they could do so naturally through exercise, without harm to their bodies, then they might choose to alter their habits. It is possible that some of society's drug problems are related to this biological enzyme deficiency, and points to why addicts find it so difficult to give up drugs.

Secondly, a decrease in demand may prompt major pharmaceutical companies to invest in other, less lucrative but essential areas of medicine. Instead of seeking to sustain profits by plastering over illness, they may look to creating real cures.

While I do not believe that all of our mental health problems can be solved by exercise, I do believe that future research will reveal that environmental pressures like emotional turmoil, job loss and stress can make it difficult to cope with life. But if we're in a positive and balanced state of mind, these issues become less challenging. Successfully dealing with barriers is all about the quality of our mental attitude – the mental 'infrastructure' we possess. Feelings of insecurity, fear and loathing should be dealt with – recovering a positive outlook on life through body management is a vital part of that process.

Although work on the complexity of the mind and its dysfunction is still in its infancy, studies that have been performed repeatedly show that exercise can improve our mental abilities and go some way towards preventing mental decline. Psychologist James Blumenthal found that the key benefits of exercise were 'above and beyond' what was expected after depression was lifted.[2]

Movement was found to affect functions controlled by specific areas of the brain: memory, organization and the ability to juggle different tasks. But attention, concentration and psycho-motor skills controlled by different parts of the brain were not affected. Why? Because, Blumenthal feels, just as exercise improves muscle tone and function, so it has a similar effect on the brain – and those parts of the brain may in fact need another type of stimulation.

If we look at the value of exercising the brain itself, studies of mental degenerative diseases like Alzheimer's and senile dementia have shown that being inactive and watching a lot of television can raise the level of brain-cell deterioration – a process that actually begins at an earlier age than was once believed. American scientists have found that our memories start to decline in our mid-twenties, at the same rate as for people in their sixties and seventies. We simply do not notice this occurring because we have more brain volume than we need. The brain, like other muscles in our body, must be used, exercised and trained to maintain mental health. For Dr Denise Park at the Centre for Ageing and Cognition, 'Cognitive performance is a direct result of brain activity and structure, much like cardiovascular fitness relates to our ability to exercise and perform physical tasks.'[3]

Finally, a Cambridge University study in 1997 showed that memory decline was closely linked to how people kept their brains stimulated.

I hope that I have managed to convince you how important movement is to your mental health.

BARRIERS TO EXERCISE

Only 20 per cent of the population regularly exercise, and not having enough time is the main excuse. It's common for us to neglect our health in favour of other activities that we deem more 'essential', but surely three hours of exercise a week out of the 168 hours available is not too much too ask – with a bit of commitment and organization you can fit it into your life. Too often we put our health on the back burner, hoping nothing too awful will go wrong while we take care of everyone else in our lives. Take control of the situation and prioritize *yourself*, too.

Working mothers or those who travel a lot find it difficult to find opportunities to exercise; on top of this their situation is often emotionally and financially complex. I really feel for mothers who suffer from a lack of support at home; they opt selflessly to put all their resources into their offspring without a thought for their own physical welfare, and find themselves exhausted at the end of a working day and guilty that they have not done more.

More people would exercise if they could get something for nothing or for very little investment. The whole point of our bodies being structured in the way they are (i.e. that they need regular movement to remain healthy) is so we make the time to learn about ourselves – it's inherently built into our life pattern.

I have also heard many stories from people concerning injuries or illnesses that prevent them working out. This is most curious because these very people tend to be fit enough to perform all kinds of other tasks, such as climbing stairs, going shopping, carrying heavy bags and standing for hours drinking and socializing – all without the need for medical attention. In the end, all they've needed is a gentle supervised programme aimed at healing the problems they have rather than opting out altogether.

Few of us actually have debilitating problems, and many ailments are actually due to a lack of exercise. For example, a large number of hours and money is lost each year through sick leave caused by back pain, yet medical consensus suggests that very few sufferers actually have conditions that warrant treatment, and would benefit from exercises that strengthen their back. Too many hours sitting on chairs with inadequate support, at the computer screen, or simply walking about with bad posture due to muscle deterioration has contributed to our nation's 'back-pain crisis'.

Being overweight, elderly or just in poor health have all been given as reasons for inactivity. Or people claim they are not the sporty type, saying, 'I need to relax – I'm too stressed-out.' Or indeed, blaming others – 'There is no one to do it with,' or 'There are no suitable facilities to use.'

None of these is a good enough excuse; they are evidence of us not being ready take control of our health.

Barriers can be removed, and are part of normal everyday life. No one ever said that life was going to be easy with everything handed to us on a plate. They are not overwhelming problems and should not be perceived as such. Whenever I watch the participants of the Para Olympics I often think how lucky I've been not to have had the challenge of a missing limb – I feel totally humbled by their achievements and the incredible tests they've overcome to be athletes. It's a big wake-up call.

Working out regularly disciplines the mind and, although it can appear to be restricting, actually creates greater freedom. Some people find it restrictive to have to be somewhere at a set time, but exercise opens and relaxes your mind so that you can perform all the other tasks in your life more easily and efficiently - so exercise time is always time well spent!

We'll now see how exercise does this by looking at two important areas of fitness: cardiovascular and strength training.

AEROBIC FITNESS

Fortunately, I've loved exercise from childhood; moving around was always my preferred leisure activity both in and after school – later it became my profession. But it was not until my early thirties that I actually explored the type of training programmes necessary to maintain optimum health. Today clients seek my skills to create workouts that will change the state of their health and lifestyle in a balanced way.

The whole point of exercise is to become fitter and healthier, and for me movement should satisfy these basic criteria to be of full benefit.

Aerobic exercise performs this task. One of the major by-products of aerobic exercise can be weight loss, but it does not necessarily follow. For instance, in London I have had many women clients who carry a high percentage of fat on their bodies in relation to their volume of muscle, even though they may only weigh 120 lb/8.5 stones.

Although these women wanted weight loss, they really needed to become fit to achieve the lean, youthful figure they desired. By lowering their overall body fat and increasing the volume of fat-free mass/muscle in the body, they achieved little to no actual weight loss but dramatically changed the internal quality of their bodies and how they looked externally. Fat weighs less than muscle, so as body fat reduced and solid muscle tissue increased, their weight stayed the same but they were healthier.

Yes, we all want to look good; it helps to motivate us to exercise – but becoming *healthy* should be your prime incentive. Setting a long-term health goal encourages us to relax into the process and forces us to abandon more superficial aims – we live in the moment as opposed to disconnecting from the whole experience of self-renewal.

To be classified as fit (according to the American College of Sports Science), we should have:

1. cardiovascular/aerobic fitness (exercise the whole body for long periods and have the circulatory and respiratory systems supply the fuel to keep moving)

2. a lean body mass (over 75 per cent of body weight that is muscle and bone)

3. the ability to use muscles without getting tired (muscular endurance)

4. strength

5. and, finally, flexibility.

All these components should be built into workouts to keep us healthy, but many people mistakenly think activities like going for walks, gardening, swimming or even yoga and golf are enough to make them fit – they are only pieces of the fitness puzzle, largely aerobically-based with little to no strength or flexibility training at amateur level. Balanced fitness programmes will, according to the World Health Organization (WHO):

- regulate blood-glucose levels and improve blood-lipid profile

- positively stimulate adrenalin and noradrenalin

- enhance sleep quality and quantity

- substantially improve all aspects of cardiovascular functioning.

Long-term benefits include:

- improved muscle strength, bone-density and increased fat-free mass

- preservation and rehabilitation of flexibility

- improved gastrointestinal transit time, as well as the prevention and slowing down of the decline in balance and co-ordination due to ageing.

These benefits are partly due to a very efficiently operating cardiovascular system through aerobic exercise – movement that uses or trains the heart, lungs and entire respiratory system to produce energy (running, cycling, swimming, cross-country skiing, step and circuit classes). The body needs to stimulate this energy system to remain healthy; illnesses like high blood pressure, strokes, obesity and heart disease are all improved with aerobic exercise.

A lack of aerobic training makes it hard for us to meet the energy demands of modern life. We become stressed from long working hours, less able to cope with emotional and financial strain, constantly feel tired and lose our ability to problem-solve, ultimately finding it difficult to relax without the aid of stimulants, which increase general irritation and frustration!

Aerobic exercise increases the volume of oxygen in our bodies by using the entire respiratory system – it becomes stronger while supporting growth and repair. A lack of dynamic physical movement encourages our bodies to create blockages if this type of deep-cleansing process is not carried out regularly in everyday life. Like driving a car at fast speed, exercise allows toxins (active in skin lymph but released in sweat and via carbon dioxide from the lungs) to be expelled from the body by shifting into top gear.

While moving, the body's need for oxygen increases and the lungs supply more oxygen to the blood. The heart will then pump more oxygenated blood to the working muscles. If the supply is not continuous, this causes an energy imbalance and the blood can become acidic (raised blood lactate), which results in fatigue or tiredness. Once tired, the body will have difficulty in sustaining high levels of physical activity. However, by taking part in aerobic exercise three to five times a week, the body is trained to produce greater amounts of energy, not only for the duration of that particular activity but for our everyday lives.

At rest, our body's oxygen intake is low, and as this energy requirement is small, our aerobic system can easily cope (i.e. operate without stress). But as the demand for energy increases, such as during the initial stages of exercise, our body can use two other energy supplies before switching to the aerobic system for long-term fuel.

The first of these is muscle glycogen (sugar) and the second a non-oxygen emergency system that can only supply fuel for a short time. The aerobic system, through its use of oxygen, fat *and* glycogen, produces energy for long periods (depending on our level of fitness). It is the energy system used in most sports, especially long-distance running, dancing, skiing, cycling, etc., and takes about six to ten minutes to become fully operational when we're exercising.

This is why it is important to have a proper warm-up period – the body needs at least ten minutes to know that it will be required to shift into long-term fuel use. The greater the demand for oxygen becomes, the more the aerobic system is used, until it totally takes over all the energy needs for exercise.

Liver glycogen is converted to glucose and released into the blood to provide fuel, and this in turn triggers the adipocytes (fat cells) to release more and more fat from the body. This process takes a further two to four minutes to become fully operational – hence, aerobic exercise must be part of the bag of effective tools for weight loss and maintenance.

Fat Insights

The main body of research into our fat cells suggests that when we gain weight our existing adipocytes (fat cells) become enlarged, filled with more lipid, which causes them to grow, rather than our making new ones. New fat cells tend to occur only in cases of extreme obesity.

Weight loss usually results in shrinkage of the fat cells but no change in their number, which is why it is so easy to put weight back on if food intake and exercise are not monitored. The cells are there already waiting to be filled up. Aerobic exercise creates effective drainage of fat cells, as it uses this fuel for energy. And although we are not all born with the same number of fat cells (research shows that there is as much as a 25 per cent variable in body-fat cells that is biologically determined), 30 per cent are dependant on cultural influences and what we eat.

How fat is processed in the body and how it functions are fascinating because these questions throw up further issues about why we should be watchful about the volume and quality of fats eaten and stored on our bodies.

Toxins are held in the fat and milk of animals that we eat – from antibiotics in non-organic cow's milk to high mercury levels in fish like tuna and swordfish. If we consume these animals, then we too will hold these harmful toxins in our body, which can potentially cause illness.

It makes sense to eat animal produce that has been organically reared to cut down on our contact with unhealthy dangerous fats.

Also, manufacturing industries like the textile and detergent businesses often use heavy metals, chlorine bleach and chlorine compounds, which have been proven to be particularly hazardous to our health. They use and dispose of large amounts of dioxins (pathogen and carcinogenic compounds) into the air and water. These dioxins, over time, get into the food chain and are stored, yet again, in our body fat. It makes sense that we should aim to keep our fat cells as toxin-free as possible.

Large fish like tuna, swordfish and marlin now inhabit polluted seas and have been found with high levels of heavy metals in their bodies. We should also check the levels of heavy metals and pollution we hold in our bodies caused by living in increasingly toxic environments.

Maintaining moderate body-fat levels is not only an issue of health or aesthetics but should form part of our weekly cleansing routine. Aerobic exercise aids this by emptying out fat cells, which reduces the effects of toxin build-up.

It's a big issue for women because our bodies carry more fat than men's and, when we have children, our breast milk could well be contaminated from our poisonous fat stores. Government healthcare for pregnant women should include tests on milk for heavy-metal build-up prior to and after birth as part of their ante-natal and post-natal health programme.

Aerobic training helps to correct metabolic imbalances by speeding up the volume of calories used not only while working out but afterwards, throughout the day. Our bodies need energy to perform basic functions like cell renewal, and to fuel the processes of the internal organs. This low-powered basic state is known as the RMR (resting metabolic rate).

If a person with a naturally low RMR works out, this increases the number of calories used. It is this increased turnover of calories that creates an improved and more efficient metabolic rate. The taller, heavier and more muscular a person, the higher the RMR tends to be.

Exercise coupled with a reduction in food intake has been proven to be the most successful way to lose excess weight, become fitter and to maintain a positive ratio of body fat to fat-free mass.

Crash dieters opt for a dramatic reduction in calories which falls well below the RMR, but this not only gets rid of fat but also lean muscle tissue and water which, in the long term, slows down the metabolic rate. It confuses the body into holding on to all resources in order to preserve energy to carry out vital functions. Very low-calorie diets slow down the speed at which food is used for energy, as the body cannot tell the difference between calorie counting and the threat of starvation, and therefore slows down into preservation mode.

The more frugal the diet, the more the body hangs on to the fat reserves, forcing cycles of having to eat less and less to sustain weight loss as the metabolic rate slows. Usually weight is piled back on as soon as normal eating is resumed because, again, the body does not know if it is still in starvation mode or whether food will be available permanently.

While a low-calorie diet may cause the loss of 500 calories a day, a workout of 400 kcal expenditure plus moderate food reduction of, say, 300 calories, can cause a 700 kcal deficit without harmful metabolic results. If you over-exercise to achieve large calorie deficits, then your body will be more prone to injury and stress, which will ultimately prohibit movement – use of either on its own is only partially beneficial to reaching your final goals.

Exercise is the only way to counteract the metabolic fallout from yo-yo dieting, as it aids a constant metabolic rate. Moderate to vigorous aerobic exercise like running, cycling, circuit and step or aerobic classes speeds up the metabolism so that fat use increases for 12–24 hours after a 90-minute session. To aid weight loss, the American College of Sports Medicine (2004) recommends we should aim to create a kcal expenditure of 300–500 kcal a day, or 1,500–2,000 kcal a week.

Furthermore, because exercise increases the number of muscle cells and reduces body fat, there should be a rise in the RMR, which should in turn cause us to need more food to live, not less. The more active tissues there are in the body in the form of muscle, the more efficient the body is at using fat for energy rather than simply storing it.

Aerobic Training – The Lowdown

To get the best out of your workout you need to ensure that you are using your cardiovascular system effectively, so I'm going to take you through what should be happening in your body.

After a ten-minute warm-up period your body should be in its 'training zone', i.e. using its aerobic energy system efficiently. The training zone reflects how much oxygen you're getting into your body, and can be measured by how fast your heart is beating – you should aim to remain in this zone for as long as possible.

During this phase you can gradually increase the intensity of the workout – but not to the extent that it causes your heart rate to suddenly climb – you should always aim to maintain a comfortable oxygen intake within the limits of this training zone. Workouts should aim to use the vital capacity of our lungs by operating within 60–85 per cent of our maximum heart rate (MHR), depending on fitness levels.

To calculate your maximum heart rate, you take the number 220 and subtract your age, then divide this number by 100 and multiply the result by 60 (or by 85, depending on whether you wan to know what 60 or 85 per cent of your MHR is).

For example, if a 30-year-old person wants to calculate 60 per cent of their MHR, the equations would be $220 - 30 = 190$, divided by $100 = 1.9$, multiplied by $60 = 114$ beats per minute. This figure represents the target for an unconditioned adult for, say, a couple of sessions. To improve fitness levels, over several sessions our 30-year-old should aim to perform between 60 and 85 per cent of their MHR – that is, their pulse rate should be kept between 114 and 161 bpm (beats per minute).

Although the heart rate is a good way of assessing the intensity of a workout, today exercise professionals believe that, for people with cardiovascular disease or co-ordination problems, or for the very overweight, the total distance and exercise duration are more effective ways of maximizing energy expenditure.

For instance, the American College of Sports Medicine now recommends 40–60 minutes of aerobic exercise at least four days a week to reduce weight. They also recommend that workouts should be regulated by *time* rather than by intensity. So, if the duration of an exercise programme is 20 minutes and 2.5 km are covered, by the end of the year, or over the next few months, 60 minutes/8 km each session should be an achievable goal.

I have found both the maximum heart rate and distance/time measurements beneficial, as both allow you to record your progress accurately and stop you settling into a comfort zone which causes your sessions to become ineffective over a period of time – doing the same exercises in the same ways reduces their value. You need to constantly stimulate your body with new movements.

Our lungs need to be progressively worked out by aerobic exercise, because their full capacity is underused but constantly challenged by environmental pollutants. We have a six-litre lung capacity, of which only half a litre is used every day and one litre keeps stored air. Our maximum air intake is four litres, and although our lungs usually hold one litre in expiratory reserves, this still leaves one litre not being used. Aerobic exercise makes us increase the use of this vital capacity to intake more air, which in turn boosts the efficiency of our whole respiratory system.

Towards the end of a hard workout some people experience fatigue that's painful due to a build-up of lactic acid in the blood. As the speed or intensity of the workout increases to provide more energy, so does the production of carbon dioxide, which can trigger the anaerobic (no-oxygen) system to supply energy for movement. The intensity of the muscle contractions causes a compression of the small arteries so that no glucose, fat or oxygen can enter the muscle cell. The body now has to take fuel from that already stored in the muscles – but usually there will be very little left, as it will already have been depleted in the initial stage of exercise.

Eventually, as more lactic acid is formed, released into the bloodstream and placed in muscle tissue, the body's ability to function efficiently aerobically is compromised, making it unable to produce adequate amounts of energy.

For most people, this process will force us to slow down, to reduce energy demand – or for the suitably trained, to rely more heavily on the anaerobic system to continue.

Lactic-acid tolerance is usually low in most of us – about 40–50 seconds – and as only a small percentage is changed back into glycogen in the liver, the majority remains in the blood and muscles. You'll know it's there when you find it difficult to breathe and suffer tiredness and a heavy feeling in your muscles, which will force you to end the workout. Lactic build-up usually occurs when the heart is accelerated to between 85 and 90 per cent of MHR.

Workouts regulated purely for the purpose of fat-burning and aerobic training should not involve the long-term use of anaerobic energy. Instead, a workout should become, in geometric terms, a curve – including a brief warm-up, a gradual increase of the heart rate to between 60 and 85 per cent of the MHR, then a gradual decrease with a cool-down, as illustrated in the diagram overleaf.

This measured way of training prepares the body to accept more positive strain, and has been invaluable in providing results for clients – either improved fitness or weight loss. After aerobic workouts the body feels invigorated, cleansed and more awake, due to the high volume of toxins released and the increased oxygen intake.

As well as a stronger heartbeat, cardiovascular training produces an increase in stroke volume (the amount of blood pumped out with each contraction), which in turn slows down the number of beats the heart has to perform per minute to push blood around the body, so easing

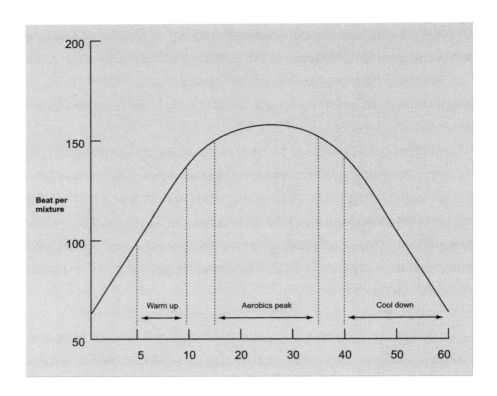

internal stress. This also helps to normalize blood pressure and increases the volume of the cells' intake of oxygen.

Although the UK government's agenda is set on getting more people to exercise, experience has led me to believe we need more education about why we are doing it and what is going on in our bodies. Here are some of the most commonly asked questions about training principles.

Will running three times a week at the same pace and distance produce the same quality of results?

No, the more skilled one becomes at any workout routine, the fewer calories are used. According to Dr Mathew Mill, this is an evolutionary trait to conserve energy to ensure survival. Exercise intensity should gradually increase over time, which not only increases the rate of calories burned at the time but also raises the metabolic rate.

Do I need to perform vigorous exercise to achieve maximum fat use?

This is still a very controversial issue within the profession, but experience directs me to answer yes, but only with certain conditions.

Many of us are still under the misconception that we can gain significant benefits from lifestyle activities such as gardening, housework and just climbing the stairs at home or work, but this is not true. These activities will not produce the health benefits of structured exercise. Research shows that moderate activities like walking produce no associated reduction in mortality or increased fitness gains.

All things being equal, a person with no stress and no physical, hormonal or emotional disabilities maximizes fat loss with intensive exercise. Exercising at around 70 per cent of maximum heart rate for 45–60 minutes causes a greater rise in resting metabolic rate, an increase in fat-burning enzymes and also acts as an appetite-suppressant.

What constitutes vigorous exercise is a relative concept. There are conditions like stress, tiredness, recovery from illness, certain medication or emotional traumas that artificially increase the heart rate. On these occasions a vigorous workout may simply be a brisk uphill walk, a game of badminton, a 30-minute swim or gardening – effective training does not need to over-stress the body.

These activities bring the body into the training zone, but once the stress is removed the heart rate will usually normalize so that the intensity of a workout needs to be positively increased. Only the intensity or duration should be increased within a single session, not both at the same time, as this creates too much stress on the body and lowers performance.

A person with no barriers needs to exercise at a higher intensity just to produce the same heart rate of 70 per cent and gain the same result as an unfit person. The fitter one becomes, the more difficult it is to achieve training-zone MHR targets.

The other reason high-intensity workouts are beneficial is that moderate exercise may burn less fat and won't deplete muscle glycogen, so that any excess energy of post-exercise meals is converted into body fat. However, if after an hour of intensive exercise, muscle glycogen is depleted, the net meals' excess energy will be directed towards refilling muscle glycogen rather than the fat stores.

Which activities are best for burning calories and effective aerobic training?

The most effective aerobic exercise, performed over an hour for a 70 kg person, has been found to be cross-country skiing, closely followed by running an average of 11.5 km using 633 kcal. Cycling (12–14 mph), circuit training, tennis (singles) and stepping all burned 563 kcal, while general aerobics, leisurely swimming and weight training all used 422 kcal.

Is aerobic exercise the best way to lose weight?

No, not on its own. I have found the combination of aerobic exercise, strength training and nutritional changes to be the most effective way to lose weight and keep it off. Continuous aerobic exercise without resistance training will only degenerate active muscle tissue, especially in the upper body, which will increase body fat and slow metabolism over a period of time. Strength training increases lean body mass and aids the metabolic rate while resting; a pound of muscle requires about 45 calories to maintain, while the same amount of body fat needs just five to six calories a day.

BUILDING MUSCLE

Preserving our strength is essential to our health and keeps us fit; we do this by placing a demand or overload on our body's muscles through weight-bearing exercise. Our muscles then adapt to this demand by becoming stronger and more able to sustain muscular energy during activity.

For example, to play tennis you need all-round fitness, but the upper part of the body would need to be particularly strong because of the nature of the sport. The stronger these muscles are, the more likely they would be able to cope with changes in the endurance level of a match. However, these gains would not necessarily be transferable to a sport like football, where the muscles of the legs would need to be more powerful than the upper body.

Working your muscular system through resistance training develops not only strength and endurance but also improves the ability of your muscles to recover more rapidly from the stress of exercise. You can do strength exercises by using your own body weight, equipment like hand weights, bands or weighted balls, or on machines like those available in gyms.

As well as helping to increase your body's metabolic rate through increased muscle mass, training with weights strengthens muscles so that the skeleton can move with ease, and enhances bone mineral density while fortifying connective tissue, ligaments and tendons.

Strong muscles support the joints they cross; inadequate strength, on the other hand – often a result of lessened support – leads to musculo-skeletal disorders that result in pain and gross discomfort like back pain. Lower back pain is just one of many disorders that causes record numbers of working days to be lost in sick leave – a situation that could be eased by increasing muscular strength in the back and stomach, which might also prevent the onset of its symptoms in the first place.

Our bone tissue works in a dynamic way, changing in density and form in response to the stresses placed upon it. A lack of exercise and low body weight can cause a rapid loss of bone mass. We cannot move our skeleton without muscle, and muscles can't thrive if there is no bone to attach to.

Our muscles act as a corset for the skeleton – protecting internal organs – which helps us to keep upright and maintain posture. We're able to straighten our shoulders and prevent our abdomen from pushing outwards, so holding up the spine and head. When toned and strong, muscles help to reduce the risk of injury.

If you persevere, training with weights builds up weak muscles so your posture improves and there's more room for internal organs to function without stress.

This dynamic yet delicate relationship between soft and hard tissues appears to have been erased from our consciousness. We've become attentive to the more superficial parts of our bodies rather than what lies beneath the skin. Muscle and bone have a finely tuned symbiotic relationship that is individually genetically determined. Each of us has our own individual code that determines how much muscle, bone and fat is on our body – some of us may need only perform minimal weight-bearing exercise to maintain health, while others will need more.

REAL STRENGTH

It is a commonly-held myth that muscle size actually determines its strength. Strength is also determined by the ability of the nervous system to activate muscles. People involved in sport such as martial arts tend to have comparatively small, densely packed muscle tissue but are as relatively strong as larger-muscled sportspeople.

Our nervous system activates muscles by sending impulses from the central nervous system via nerve cells called motor neurons, which are embedded within all muscle tissue. These neurons, when grouped together in muscle fibre, are called motor units. The amount of force created when a muscle contracts depends on the number of motor units that are fired and the number of times this process is repeated.

Resistance training stimulates an increase in the number of motor units used at any given time and quickens the speed at which they are fired. This in turn increases the efficiency of the nervous system's drive to muscle, and clears any blocks in nerve pathways – their communication and function are greatly improved. The more muscles are used, the more efficiently they respond to the nervous system, which creates a more effective muscular system. And improved co-ordination within the muscular system allows for the production of greater force – that is, makes us stronger.

These nervous-system gains have to take place before changes like an increase in muscle size can be seen. It explains why in the early stages of training, although you may feel stronger, you may not necessarily see results for at least two months. In this way, strength is partially created from the repeated demand put onto muscles to generate force. If this demand is not raised through exercise, the body will become weaker over time – so if you don't use it, you will lose your strength.

Nowadays controversy rages over exactly what causes muscle growth. Is it due to an increase in the individual muscle fibres or due to the entire muscle tissue getting larger? Recent studies dismiss the theory of increased muscle fibre, as this is largely genetically pre-set; rather, evidence suggests that it is the whole muscle tissue that grows. The degree to which growth can occur depends on several factors.

Muscles are made up of two fibres: slow twitch (these are oxidative and have a high aerobic capacity for endurance actives) and fast twitch (glycolytic and best suited to activities that require strength, speed and power). Gaining strength and size usually takes place in the fast-twitch fibre, even though progressive weight training will promote development of both fast and slow types of fibre.

No amount of resistance training can increase the number of fast-twitch fibres. People born with greater numbers of slow-twitch fibres can only increase the working capacity of the fast-twitch fibres they already possess. Therefore, to a large extent the potential for increased muscle growth and strength is genetically pre-set by the number of fast-twitch fibres that already exist.

Diet and the ability of muscles to synthesize protein also play important roles, but there is no consensus about why this is so.

Nutritionists argue that high levels of protein consumption do not aid muscle growth, while body-builders advocate the opposite. Though in the case of the average person excessive protein consumption is converted to fat, for those with increased muscle-fibre activity (created through manual work, sport or exercise) this is not the case. Their greater protein uptake is used directly to provide energy for labour-intensive work.

One explanation is that fast-twitch fibres increase in size through combining with protein, while slow-twitch fibres develop by the slow breakdown of protein. Hence, those adults working at building their fast-twitch fibres may need to consume more dietary protein and its amino acids (the building blocks of muscle tissue.)

Training assists this process by creating tension that provides a signal, which is read by the genetic machinery of the cell. This stimulates protein integration. No growth will occur if training is at too low an intensity – during training, part of the muscle must be broken down, which causes it to be repaired gradually at a denser level, to adapt to the increased overload. This skeletal muscle damage following heavy resistance exercise is not detrimental but makes our bodies stronger.

LET'S TALK AGE AND GENDER

You may have gathered by now that aerobic training is only a part of the weight-loss, health and exercise story – nutrition and resistance training have important roles, too.

Many of us, especially women, are not aware of the major role active muscle plays in our body. Somehow it remains a mystery. No matter how many reports show the escalation of degenerative diseases like osteoporosis, back pain and joint decay, the connection to a lack of resistance exercise is rarely made.

Although our society is youth-obsessed, few of us attempt to maintain the youth and health of our bodies naturally with weight training or sport. With adequate, safe training techniques we can secure and prepare our bodies for a fit old age. I'll take it for granted that you want to live out your senior years free from pain and not suffer from illnesses that compromise your independence.

We women need to do more weight-bearing exercise to remain healthy, but often face confusing and extreme information. Bombarded with images of either incredibly thin or high-body-fat women in the media, we're unsure of how our bodies *should* look or be maintained for health. Too much store is put in myths that strength training creates masculine bodies – a feat that is quite difficult without serious time commitment and a little testosterone. We have become fearful of having a strong muscular system because it simply is not in fashion. Many choose solely to burn fat with excessive aerobic exercise – a process that can increase the risk of injury. We need weight training to increase our metabolic rate.

Lean, toned muscle is youthful. Men are ahead of the ageing game by virtue of the fact that their bodies carry more muscle (around 42 per cent) with only 12–14 per cent body fat, so they need to eat more to feed their muscle mass. I feel passionately that strength training for women is a necessity because, coupled with aerobic training, it really helps us to regulate our sometimes challenging body-fat levels (which should be around the 20–25 per cent mark). Even in our outward-appearance-fixated society, weight training will naturally help you to change the way you look, often correcting muscular imbalances while increasing your ability to cope with the physical demands of modern life – a package I don't think many cosmetic surgeons can offer.

Mainstream images of women's bodies do not show healthy musculature, and if the average woman compares or tries to emulate these images, it will compromise her health. Such fashion, beauty, film and advertising images should be seen as the fantasy and illusion that they are – an idealization and not the reality. Muscle creates shape on our bodies, and when destroyed or dying makes our bodies appear flat and underdeveloped.

Likewise, resistance training should not only be pursued as an end in itself but as the counterbalance and stabilizing force to aerobic activity. It provides an essential service to our bodies when nature begins to withdraw her gifts. We start to age in our late twenties – it is believed that the body produces liberal amounts of growth hormone until this time and then stops, after which we're on the path to decline.

This is why it's so important for young people to have plenty of exercise – we need to invest in our bodies for the rainy day (old age) when we won't have this special helping hand from nature.

Our lack of exercise tends not to show until our early thirties, but these days this is all changing with childhood and teenage obesity figures rising every year. Yes, we've all seen manifest thickened waistlines and increased levels of tiredness, and people generally feeling more stressed-out at the slightest thing. By this age we will have been without nature's helper – growth hormone – for as much as five years, and as a result our muscular system would have been getting weaker and weaker.

Ageing creates a slowing down in the rate at which the body regenerates and repairs, but training helps to increase and maintain the renewal process. With the appropriate weights programme it is possible to maintain the muscle tone of a youthful body in middle age – which does not mean that time has somehow stopped but simply that this process has been slowed.

Without weight training we lose around one pound of muscle every two years. An example made famous by Wayne Westcott is that a 40-year-old woman who weighs the same as she did in college has replaced 10 pounds of muscle with 10 pounds of fat due to natural ageing, which accounts for a big difference in body composition.

Muscle tissue has high-energy requirements in order to live and repair, and which raise our overall metabolic rate. Every pound of muscle gained raises the metabolic rate by 50 calories a day, while every pound lost lowers it by 50 calories a day. It is a myth that constantly depleting the body's fat reserves and dieting will achieve the appearance of youth so desired in our culture – keeping your tissue alive by eating healthily and using it will.

Consider this: if two adults both eat 2,000 calories a day, after ten years the one with no resistance programme will have lost 5 pounds of muscle and will need to eat 250 fewer calories in order not to gain weight. The one following a resistance programme will have gained two pounds of muscle and can consume 2,100 calories a day without gaining any weight. Developing muscle tissue helps women to control their body-fat levels without being at the mercy of the diet industry.

THE GYM

Traditionally, structured exercise programmes should develop skills that test balance, co-ordination, agility, speed and the ability to react to stimulation – gyms easily help you to fulfil these criteria. This is not to say that other forms of exercise are irrelevant, but that gyms help you to maintain all the components of fitness with ease – they are a good option.

Gyms have been unduly criticized for being boring due to the repetitive nature of structured programmes, and many initially avid gym-goers have failed to achieve their dreams of sportsmanship. But let's clear up this confusion. If we look at the sports many of us admire, a lot of work goes on behind the scenes.

Most if not all professional athletes and sportspeople spend hours training in the gym, performing those repetitive movements to finely tune their body's responses – physical growth and health are necessary for high-performance results.

Footballers, swimmers, sprinters, cyclists and squash players not only play their sport but require advanced dietary advice, equipment and a great amount of technology to allow them to compete. It is on the pitch, in the pool or indeed while climbing mountains that all the components of fitness are tested and merge together to produce a successful performance.

Structured training like that offered in gyms prepares us for a more active life, so that the specific training and stamina needed for swimming, badminton, roller skating, country walks or even the speed of everyday life are available to us.

Gyms give you more control over your time, as you work out at a time that is suitable for your lifestyle. Training tends to be non-competitive in the sense that your exercise programme does not involve issues of winning or losing. And because exercise programmes are made solely to suit your individual needs, they are more effective at achieving results quickly. Classes offer general exercises with few variables, designed for a group of mixed abilities.

I view going to the gym in the same way as going to the supermarket – I have to attend to gain the greater benefit of being able to heal and maintain my body. It is the safest, cheapest, most convenient and effective preventative health-plan I can invest in.

Gym exercises try to emulate and test muscle contraction through a full range of joint movement – moves that may rarely take place in everyday life but which are essential to balancing muscle tissue in the body.

For the beginner, after body-weight exercises, machines are the easiest way to learn how to isolate major muscles; they are safe and simple to use, as the weights are contained in a fixed frame – if dropped, there is a low risk of injury. The level of skill required is not high (it's not rocket science), allowing for the relationship between the motor units and muscle fibre to become established before progressing onto more sophisticated exercises.

Machines reduce a lot of the hassle of training, such as waiting for bars and weights to be free, as well as the need for a partner to guide you through an exercise safely, which can be a chore. But sole use of machines will not provide total muscular development because, once your muscles have mastered a particular move, gains begin to diminish unless greater stimulation is provided.

As a result, free-weight exercises are usually mixed into weights programmes, as they provide variety and you're not restricted to a fixed arc of movement. They require more skill, concentration and technique, as the joint cycles at which the muscles work can be raised. For example, a bicep curl can be performed with a single weighted bar, over a bench or seated on an incline with dumbbells.

With as little as two hours' a week commitment and rest, strength training can provide great results. Although some people prefer to train different muscles on different days, rest allows muscles to recover adequately from tears within the fibres. If a workout is performed and progressed slowly, the effect of this damage is hardly noticeable, but some people try to do too much, resulting in pain. Recovery usually takes 24–48 hours, from which worked muscles will emerge stronger – a rest just means doing another activity like cardiovascular training.

Good movement quality is the heart of a great workout. Each set of repetitions should be performed to failure (until the action cannot be repeated) to achieve the best results in a short time frame.

Poor technique serves only to continue muscular imbalances and raise the risk of injury. And yes, training can be repetitive, but the boredom factor can be lowered by using different techniques and by gaining more knowledge about the wide range of exercises available to each and every muscle in isolation, or worked in groups, in your body – it's fascinating!

Don't perform the same workout week after week or month after month – it's not only demotivating but stops your body developing. As with the mind, change creates growth.

Factors that Affect Your Performance

Several factors will affect how you feel when you exercise, and can influence how well you perform. Sometimes you'll want to give 100 per cent but it may not always be possible – listen to your body and its limits. General fatigue, the time of day you choose to work out (apparently mid-morning or early afternoon are the best), humidity and excessive heat all increase your heart rate artificially, which will cause you to lower your workout intensity. Exercising in the cold can make a workout feel easier, so this may be an opportunity to work at a higher intensity.

Undigested food in the stomach greatly affects whether a workout can be completed successfully or not. You should eat food at least two hours prior to a session to allow your body's digestive system time to break it down and produce fuel in the blood without difficulty. If you eat too soon before a bout of exercise, your body will want to throw the food out of the stomach so that blood can be supplied to working muscles instead of to breaking down food. A tight pain in the lower stomach or 'stitch' often results, which is the body forcing a slow down and finally halting the session as it cannot supply energy for both activities. Simple sugars like fruit, rice or potatoes are usually tolerated much better than proteins, which can take up to four hours for your body to break down.

On the nutrition front, it is never a wise choice to make a heavy physical demand on the body with very little fuel. Without any or the right type of fuel you cannot expect peak performance – it's like trying to drive a car on diesel instead of the four-star petrol it needs to operate at optimum levels. And because the breakdown of proteins and fats is complex, it is necessary to understand which are the appropriate foods to eat before a workout.

Smokers who want to become fit are giving themselves a very tough time if they're unwilling to give up their habit. Smoking degenerates lung function and capacity, so workouts will feel more difficult than for non-smokers. Smoking detracts from the lung capacity available for oxygen; air ducts become blocked with nicotine, causing additional breathing difficulties.

Luckily I have never felt the need to preach to smokers about giving up – the pains in their chest when working out always seem to provide them with enough evidence to quit. Similarly, an alcohol-fuelled night out will anaesthetize the body's response to stimulation and weaken co-ordination. Any form of movement can become challenging, together with blurred vision and dehydration; all of which increases the probability of injury as well as of very poor performance.

Long before the studies were published about the length of time alcohol stays in the blood, it was common knowledge in my aerobic class. As soon as we started sweating you could smell those who had been on the amber nectar the night before – brewery-like fumes filled the air as our bodies finally broke down and got rid of excess toxins, but we felt really clean and fresh from the inside out afterwards!

However, the most beneficial aid to workouts has to be music; it helps to ease you into a session, relieves stress from the workout and also helps to move you out of one mental or emotional space into another, more harmonious environment, which promotes relaxation.

We all have favourite tracks that make us want to get up and sing and dance – the process of moving is not half as challenging if you hear music you enjoy. Fast-paced music with a heavy beat stimulates the heart to beat faster and increase blood flow around the body.

Music can hypnotize you into feeling good and into making your workout pleasurable because it makes you forget the lethargy and fatigue that often plague our bodies and, like the effects that have been noted of Mozart's music on children, it improves our cognitive function and the ability of our bodies to work in a synchronized way.

While music will not increase the intensity of the workout, it will extend your ability to tolerate and endure a workout for longer. Carefully organized music will focus your attention so that the probability of becoming bored is reduced; this in itself will delay your mind's response to your body's messages of pain or tiredness – especially when you're not feeling 100 per cent.

My clients are willing to be pushed harder if they have the right tracks lined up for when they hit the most difficult part of the workout. And by putting in this effort they feel that the workout is more productive, having achieved the maximum output possible for them. Also, in an unsatisfactory environment music can trigger pleasant emotions, which contribute to creating a pleasant working environment – a feature well documented by many psychologists and music therapists.

It is equally important to choose music that is right for you and reflects your personal taste. Many a client has reacted negatively to being in a space with very aggressive music that has 'grated on their nerves', making the workout uncomfortable. Music should have the reverse effect and even help the cool-down period at the end of the workout so much that you feel more relaxed than at the start of the session.

The only time I would not advise using headphones is when exercising in busy urban areas when you need to remain vigilant to hear possible dangers from people or traffic.

While on the subject of environment, again I would argue that natural light is incredibly beneficial to how you feel in and after a workout. It is difficult enough to find the right space to work out in, but if you are stressed about working out in a dark, unclean building, the benefits of the whole process are lessened.

Here in Britain we have growing numbers of adults who become depressed in the autumn and winter months, due to the lack of light thanks to day after day of grey cloudy weather – which has been clinically diagnosed as SAD (seasonal affective disorder). Being in natural light makes you feel more positive, which I'm sure contributes to more people being more upbeat in spring, and more willing to change their lifestyle and lose weight for the summer.

Finding the Right Gym

Finding the gym that is right for you can be a laborious and expensive task, so to take the strain out of the process I've devised a checklist of things to look out for before you part company with your cash.

1. Decide whether you want a gym with all the frills or one offering just decent equipment. You can find one offering both, but the cost tends to increase in accordance with the volume of facilities on offer, such as swimming pools, restaurants, steam rooms, hairdressers or beauty therapists. Remember that the goal is to work out and your gym will need to offer a fitness room with exercise machines, free weights, a stretching area and at least one studio for classes.

2. Try to find a gym that is easy to get to, preferably near to your home or work.

3. Membership prices vary greatly, so ask about any special offers when joining, like two people joining for the price of one, as this may be cheaper than listed prices.

4. Check what is included in the price or if there are additional charges for classes, using courts for racquet sports, or for sunbeds.

5. Many gyms offer a free visit for you to get an idea of the atmosphere. Try to make this visit at the time you are most likely to be exercising to see the gym's unique climate. Day and evening workout times are generally hugely different and you'll need to be sure that you are comfortable, whatever the environment.

PRE-WORKOUT PREP

Before you start any programme you will have to assess your fitness levels as well as make sure that your exercise experience will be as comfortable and productive as possible.

Training Shoes

Earlier in this book I talked about the need to prepare your body for exercise by making sure it can perform without pain. One of the main sites on the body to get this balance right is in your feet – the right shoes will make all the difference to the quality of your workout. Any activity that involves impact going through the body, like running, jumping, etc., will need appropriate cushioning.

Running shoes tend to be great all-rounders for up and down movements like jogging, stair-climbing, stationary biking and weight training, but they are not suitable for dance, stretching or normal cycling.

Besides needing to know whether your feet are classified as either a broad or narrow fitting, you will also need to find out the condition of your arch to get the correct fit of trainer.

If you step on to a piece of paper with a wet foot, the imprint you leave will tell you a lot. A full image (i.e. an imprint of the whole flat of your foot) indicates a tendency to over-pronate, which means that you land on the inside of your foot. You will need shoes with a firm control to prevent excess motion.

If you produce a curvy incomplete print you are probably under-pronating, which means you land on the outside of your foot. Your trainers will need to be cushioned with a firm heel and flexible forefoot.

A medium arch, which is the most common foot, requires shoes that are soft and flexible.

Another quick way to find out if you over- or under-pronate is to look at the heels of your shoes: if the heel is worn mainly on the inside at the back then your feet are likely to be flat; if they are worn on the outside you have high arches.

If your trainers do not provide adequate support, then you may need to have specially-designed insoles. These are usually made by podiatrists.

Heart-rate Monitors

As part of your workout there will be an aerobic component for your heart and lungs. To measure the intensity of the workout you will need to monitor your heart rate or your pulse. This will tell you if you are hitting your target heart rate while exercising, which in turn helps your workout to be productive and safe. As mentioned earlier, exercising at too low an intensity means that you'll not gain all the necessary health benefits, while over-exercising can strain the body and cause excessive tiredness or even injury. I've often noticed that beginners attempt to do too much initially, which causes them to drop out as they feel the workouts are too draining.

Heart-rate monitors give you an accurate reading of what your pulse is while performing. They are very easy to use.

To find out your maximum heart rate, subtract your age from the number 220. In my experience a good target heart rate to aim for is 70–80 per cent of your maximum. To find that figure, simply divide your maximum heart rate by 10 and then multiply this number by 70 for the low end of your target heart rate and by 80 for the top end. For a 35-year-old woman this figure would be 185 divided by 10 (1.85) times 70 = 129 beats per minute; multiplied by 80 we get 148 beats per minute for the top end.

It is important to remember that when performing aerobic exercise you must warm up and gradually increase the intensity of the workout to achieve the target heart rate, followed by a short cool-down.

It may take as long as 12 minutes to build up to your target heart rate, and you need to stay in this zone for as long as possible, therefore your aerobic workout should in total take at least 35–40 minutes, including three to five minutes' cool-down period.

Some people prefer to take their pulse manually during a workout. To do this you can place two fingers on the inside of your wrist, then count your heartbeat for 30 seconds. Double this figure to get the beats per minute. However, remember that this method is not as accurate as the monitor because you will have to stop exercising to take your pulse, causing your heart rate to fall.

Gym-kit Essentials

Listed below are the essential items you'll need to take with you in a kit bag to the gym. Purchase a bag large enough to carry all your equipment to the gym, which can be kept packed for whenever you feel like working out. In this bag you will need:

- a towel for the shower or to wipe down machinery after use

- hairband, heart-rate monitor, cassettes/personal stereo and a few coins for the lockers

- plastic bag for wet workout clothes and toiletries such as shampoo and body lotion; shower shoes to protect your feet from bacteria

- bottled water to help you stay hydrated during and after working out

- clothing options for both warm and cooler gym temperatures; these may include shorts, jogging bottoms, long sleeve T-shirts or tank tops and additional underwear and socks for after the workout

- post-workout healthy snacks like fruit to help prevent you buying junk food on the way home

- a fitness diary – this will help you plan your programmes prior to exercise, and monitor your progress. It can be updated immediately after the workout. Record the results of your fitness assessment, goals or what you eat daily – be honest.

KNOW YOUR BODY

You have now arrived at the stage where you'll need to find out a bit more about the condition of your body before starting your exercise programme. This is so you can get into the habit of recording your sessions, ensuring that you exercise at a level that is right for you, and accurately gauging your progress over the next three months.

Weight

By looking at your weight in comparison to your height, you get an approximate indication of how much of your body is fat and how much is dense tissue (bones, muscle, etc.). This figure is calculated using the Body Mass Index. To calculate this manually, simply divide your weight in kilograms by your height in metres squared. For example, if you weigh

63 kg and are 163 cm tall, your BMI is 23 (1.63 x 1.63 = 2.65; 63 divided by 2.65 = 23). Refer to the diagram below to see how you shape up.

Remember that your weight is dependent on many factors like genes, body type, age and gender. The BMI is also *not* an accurate measure for athletes, pregnant women or sedentary elderly people.

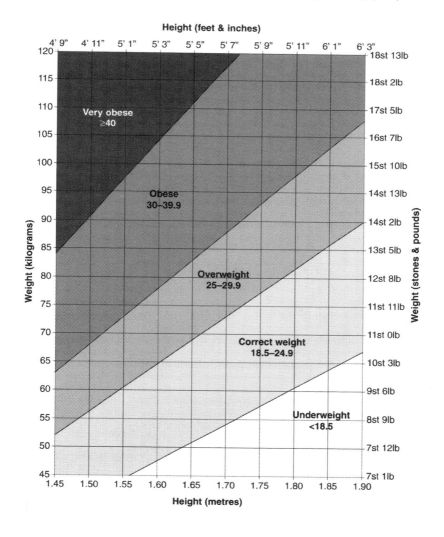

Upper-body Strength – Press-ups and Crunches

Press-ups

Get into a half press-up position (for women this means on all fours initially). Your hands should be placed directly under your shoulders, with your fingers facing forward. Do not allow your stomach to fall or arch your back. Do as many press-ups as you can in one minute.

If you manage fewer than 6, your upper body strength is poor, 7–14 is fair, 15–40 is good and anything over is excellent for women. For men, fewer than 14 is poor, 15–28 fair, 29–44 good and more than 45 excellent.

Crunches

Lie on your back with your knees bent and your hands behind your head (just the fingertips touching your head). Lift your upper body so that your head, chest and shoulder blades are off the floor but your lower back remains in contact with the floor. Lower. Do not pull on your neck. This is one crunch; you should do as many as you can in one minute without pausing.

For women, fewer than 7 is poor; 8–15 is fair, 16–35, average, 36–40 good and 40+ excellent. For men, fewer than 15 is poor, 16–20 fair, 21–40 average, 41–55 good, with excellent at 56+.

Cardiovascular Fitness

Time yourself walking one mile on a flat surface on a pre-measured route.

If you finish in fewer than 20 minutes, top marks and a good show of power-walking; 20–25 minutes indicates a good level of fitness; 25–35 minutes is average. But anything over 35 minutes, especially if you finished the route breathless, means that you need to improve your fitness levels greatly.

Flexibility

It's important that you warm up with a short walk or cycle before you start this test. Stand with your feet shoulder-width apart, bend at the waist and reach towards the floor without bending your knees. Try this a few times and record your longest reach.

You have good flexibility if you easily touch the floor, moderate if you reach your toes, but you need to work at your flexibility if you could touch neither.

Now that you've assessed how fit you are, it's time to think about setting some goals to help you keep focused. Short- and long-term goals help to keep you on track – but be realistic, as reaching for the impossible will increase the likelihood of failure.

EATING TO HELP EXERCISE

Exercise and healthy eating go hand in hand, and in Chapter 3 we covered some simple rules to help you along this route. Eating well will enhance the benefits of any exercise programme, and here I'd like to add a few more tips that directly relate to working out.

1. If you work out in the morning, eat at least one-and-a-half hours before you start and try not to eat heavy proteins that take a long time to digest. A fruit-based smoothie (blueberry, strawberry or banana), fruit salad with yoghurt and pumpkin seeds will be enough.

2. Save the heavier, slow-burning carbohydrates for after your workout. These should be low-sugar breakfast cereals like porridge, baked beans on wholemeal toast, or boiled eggs on toast. This will accelerate your metabolism further and the proteins will aid muscle regeneration.

3. If exercising at the end of the day you may feel tired and sluggish from a day at work, so you will need an energy boost from your food. This is best achieved at lunch time by eating a balanced meal of vegetables (broccoli, green beans and salad), protein (fish, chicken and tofu) and a small portion of brown rice/chickpeas/low-fat pasta. Remember to eat at least two hours before your workout.

4. To keep your metabolism high after your workout, at the end of the day be sure to eat a small meal containing protein with essential fatty acids like those in grilled salmon, trout or herring, combined with simple carbs like quinoa, sweet potatoes, green peas, vegetable soup or butter beans.

5. In between these small meals you can also eat a couple of snacks like a handful of unsalted nuts, brown rice cakes with low-fat hummus, vegetable sticks or fruit.

6. Be sure to drink plenty of water, both before and after working out, as dehydration can cause headaches, dry skin and constipation

– not to mention making your muscles feel sore and tired during the workout.

WORKOUT PROGRAMMES

These workouts are designed for those who have never exercised, those who exercise irregularly or adults looking for a whole-body training method; they will take you through a ten-week programme of progressive training. The gym is ideal for starting a movement programme as it provides variety of equipment, a social scene and, come rain or shine, as long as you have set the time aside, you'll be able to exercise in a beneficial way.

If you feel like a change from a machine-based workout, many gyms offer instructor-led classes that will fine-tune your body further, such as those offered in step aerobics, circuit, Pilates, yoga and spinning sessions.

Each workout will consist of a warm-up, aerobic and/or strength exercises, finishing with cool-down stretches. Ideally you should aim to work out three times a week to change your fitness status or to lose weight.

If you are on medication, suffer from back problems or other medical conditions, consult your doctor or health practitioner before you start these programmes.

Warm-up

Warming up the body means simply raising body temperature and warming the muscles for intense movement. Many beginners neglect this crucial start to a workout and increase their risk of strain; it's important because cold muscles are easily injured due to a lack of flexibility. All you need is five to ten minutes of brisk walking, jogging or light cycling.

Aerobic Equipment

Apart from aerobic classes, the gym offers a range of machines that work your aerobic system. Most equipment is designed to imitate activities like running, biking or skiing, but in a climate-controlled environment. You can make your workout as easy or challenging as you feel, as the equipment has manual or programmed settings to suit your mood. It is best to try them first to see which suit your body.

Although cardio machines measure heart rates and calories, use these with caution as they are not always accurate: leaning on the handlebars to take a reading will lead to a fall in the heart rate and the volume of calories used. Generally, as a rule, try never to lean over on the handlebars or consoles of exercise equipment. If the workout is too tough, lower the intensity or speed.

Having said this, the monitors on exercise machines are good for recording the length of time you want to exercise, the distance, speed and incline or resistance level.

Listed below are the machines that can be used in the aerobic part of your workout.

Stationary Bike

Upright bikes allow you to cycle on the flat or up and down hills, as if riding a regular bike.

Adjust the seat before you get on so that your knee is not completely straight when the pedal is pressed all the way down. Too high a seat will over-extend the knee; too low will shorten the full range of motion from the knee to hip. The resistance level can be increased according to the level of workout, speed or using the hill/race programmes.

Treadmill

These were created to work the heart and lungs by walking or running – brilliant if the weather is poor outside. They are also good if you are worried about impact stress on your knees or back as they have great in-built shock absorbers.

The belt can be adjusted to any speed from slow walk to sprinting. It's best to start on a slow walk until you are used to operating the machine. Also, you can adjust the gradient to make it feel as if you're walking up hills or hiking. Usually there are hand rails to help you balance when coming on or off the belt, but do not hold these when exercising.

Try to use the treadmill as if you were outside, keeping your back straight with elbows close to the body but relaxed.

Step Machine

Sometimes these are called 'Stair Master' after the popular brand found in many gyms. They use your lower body as if you were climbing stairs. Both speed and pedal resistance can be adjusted on both the manual and hill programmes.

To use, put your feet on the pedals and move them as if you were climbing stairs. Stand upright and do not lean over the rails.

Elliptical Cross Trainer

These machines are fairly new to gyms and are very good because you can burn calories as if you are jogging but with a lot less stress on the joints; also, they feel a lot easier than running. Some machines also work the upper body, as they have movable handlebars that help you to use more calories.

As with the step machine, you put your feet on the pedals and, as your feet move, they make an elliptical orbit. The size of this orbit and resistance level can be adjusted, as well as whether you move forward or backward.

Cool-down

Remember that towards the end of your cardio workout you will need to slow down your heart rate gradually. Stopping suddenly in your target heart zone can cause dizziness. I would suggest that you use the final three to five minutes of your workout to bring your heart rate down by continuing the activity but at a slower pace, just like you did in the warm-up; many machine programmes have built-in cool-downs.

Resistance Exercises

This section of your workout can be performed after a warm-up or when you've completed the cardio section. These exercises are designed to work all the major muscle groups and help you develop a greater sense of body awareness. Resistance training tends to tone women's bodies, while men tend to develop larger and heavier muscles.

As a beginner your aim is to start with a light to medium weight that you can lift for 12–15 repetitions (a rep is one full range of motion) for one or two sets. If you find that you cannot control the weight beyond eight reps, this weight is too heavy and you should try something lighter. If on completing your set it feels easy, then increase the weight for a further set.

To start you will use light weights with a high number of reps to tone and improve your endurance, but as you progress, lowering the reps (five to eight) while using a heavier weight will increase your strength. Make sure you rest for about a minute between each set.

For muscle growth and improved strength, reps of 8–12 for three sets is enough, but the weight must be heavy enough to cause muscle fatigue – that is, you must feel as though you cannot lift it for another rep. Once this process becomes easy, it is time to increase the weight.

How you perform these exercises is very important – excellent form is required for weight training, to avoid injury or, for what is more commonly the case, not getting the results you seek due to poor movement performance.

A few tips for good form are:

- Keep your spine straight and relaxed.

- Never use momentum to swing the weight. Always use slow, controlled movements, both on the way up and on the way down.

- Breathe naturally during the exercise – do not hold your breath. Breathing normally makes it easier to lift the weight and focuses your mind.

- Perform a complete range of movement.

- Do not forget to stretch afterwards.

Stretches

Towards the end of your workout, once your body is well warmed up, this is the ideal time to stretch. Stretching is just as important as the other elements of your workout. It helps to reduce post-workout soreness and muscle tension, which will make your body feel more relaxed.

Below are some simple stretches for the end of your workout. They can all be performed standing unless stated otherwise.

Calf (back of lower leg)

Lean on a wall with your forearms outstretched, place one foot behind the other, keeping the front leg bent and back leg straight, heel touching the floor. Move your hips forward, keeping your back heel on the floor, toes pointing straight ahead. Hold for 15–25 seconds, breathing deeply. Repeat on opposite leg.

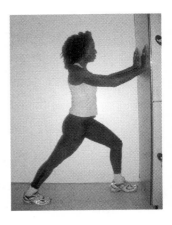

Quadriceps (front of thigh)

Using a wall for support, reach back with the right hand and grasp the right ankle and move it towards the buttocks. Stand straight with hips tilted slightly forward, knees together, slightly bent, shoulders relaxed.

You should feel the stretch in the front of your right thigh; hold for 15–30 seconds breathing in and out for a count of four beats. Repeat on opposite leg.

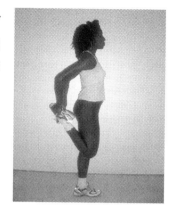

Hamstring (back of thigh)

Lie on your back and raise your left leg straight above you, keeping your right leg flat on the floor. Lower your leg. Place your hands behind the left knee and slowly pull it towards your chest to feel the stretch at the back of

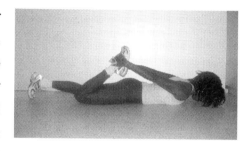

your thigh. Hold for 30 seconds, breathe deeply, then change sides.

Squats

Place feet hip-width apart with your toes pointed forward or turned out slightly. Bend your knees until they are parallel with your hips, as if sitting on a chair, tail bone pointing down, and extend your arms to shoulder level for balance. Do not drop your hips below your knees, as this will push them over your toes.

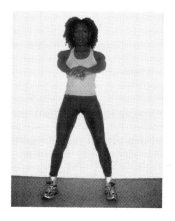

Keep your abs tight and come back up without locking out the knee joint, but squeeze your bottom muscles tight on the upward phase. Remember to breathe normally.

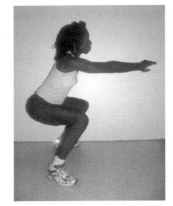

Chest

Grasp hands behind your back and lower your shoulders. Keeping your elbows and knees slightly bent, gently raise your arms upwards. You should feel the stretch in your arms, chest and shoulders. Hold for 20 seconds, breathing normally.

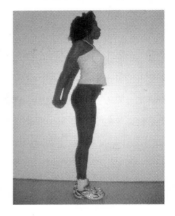

Back

Clasp your hands in front of you at shoulder height, palms facing outwards. Relax your shoulders. Keeping your elbows and knees slightly bent, feel the stretch in the middle of your upper back, shoulders and hands. Hold for 20 seconds.

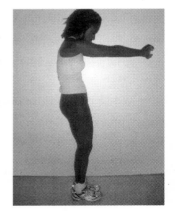

Triceps (back of upper arm) and shoulder

Place your left hand on your right shoulder with the elbow up, parallel to the floor. Use the right hand to apply gentle pressure above the left elbow, gently pressing it towards the body to feel the stretch from the back of the arm and across the right shoulder. Hold for 20 seconds, then switch arms.

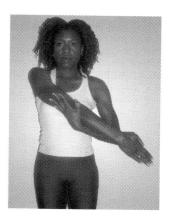

Bicep (front of upper arm)

Stand with legs hip-distance apart, knees bent. Circle your arms around the front of your body slowly four times, breathing deeply.

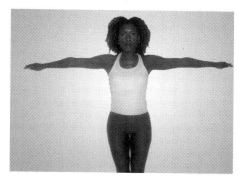
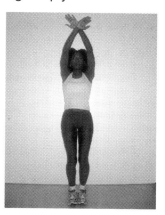

Your Workout

Now we are ready to bring all these parts together in the form of a workout.

If your goal is to lose weight, do programme B twice a week. Otherwise, simply alternate between programmes A and B for the first four weeks.

The weeks stated are only a guide; you do not have to move on to a different programme until you can perform the exercises easily with excellent form.

You'll notice that each programme has three parts – Cardio, Resistance and Stretching. It is important that you complete all three sections to ensure your body has a whole workout, and that you perform your workout in the order given.

Programme A: Weeks 1–5

Cardio	10 mins bike warm-up
	15 mins walk/jog on treadmill (MHR 60–70 per cent)
	5 mins cool-down – reduce speed or intensity
Resistance	(Exercise instructions follow, below.)
Legs:	Squats
	Standing Calf Raises
Back:	Single Arm Row
Chest:	Press-ups
Shoulders:	Overhead Press (dumbbell)
Arms:	Bicep Curl (dumbbell)
	Triceps Dips (chair or bench)
Abdominal:	Pelvic Tilts
	Crunches
Stretches	Calf, Hamstring, Quads, Shoulders, Back, Chest, Bicep, Triceps

Exercise Instructions: Weeks 1–5

a) *Squats:* Place feet hip-width apart with your toes pointed forward or turned out slightly. Bend your knees until they are parallel with your hips, as if sitting on a chair, tail bone pointing down, and extend your arms to shoulder level for balance. Do not drop your hips below your knees, as this will push them over your toes. Keep your abs tight and come back up without locking the knee joint, squeezing your bottom muscles tight on the upward phase. Remember to breathe normally. Repeat x 20 (see page 161).

b) *Standing Calf Raises:* On a platform of about 3in/8cm high (e.g. the bottom of the stairs), stand with your arms straight down by your sides. Feet hip-distance apart, start with your heels on the ground and lift your body to the point where you are standing on your toes. Hold the contraction briefly, then slowly lower your heel to the starting position. Do not bounce, as the only movement should be at the ankle joint. Keep abs firm and breathe normally. Repeat x 20.

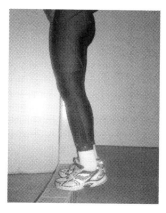

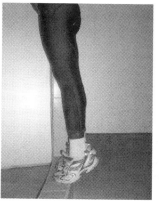

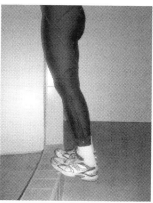

c) *Single Arm Row:* Place your left knee on a bench with your left hip directly over it. The knee of the right leg should be at about the same height and slightly bent. Put your left hand on the front edge of the bench with your fingers curled over the top. As your upper

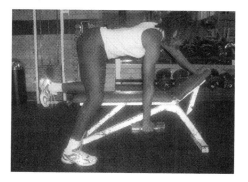

body is now parallel to floor, the dumbbell should be on the floor near your right foot. Lower your body to pick up the weight and return to this start position with your right arm hanging straight down. Lift the weight, keeping your wrist straight towards your shoulder, rotating the elbow inwards, towards your side.

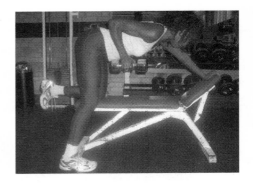

Your upper arm should be parallel to the floor or higher so that your elbow forms a right angle. To support your lower back, keep your abs firm. Pause and return the weight to the starting position. Repeat x 15.

d) *Press-ups:* You can either adopt the traditional press-up position, or those with less upper-body strength can go onto their hands and knees. Move forward so that your weight is not resting directly on your kneecaps, at slightly more than a 90-degree angle, feet in the air or on the floor. Bend your arms and slowly lower your chest to within 2in/5cm of the floor. Exhale as you straighten your arms and return to the starting position. Lift and lower your body as a single unit; do not allow your back to arch or stomach to sag. Repeat x 15.

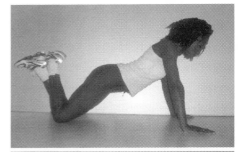

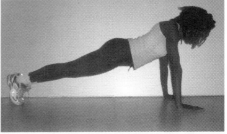

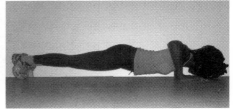

e) Overhead Press: Stand with feet shoulder-width apart, holding your weights with your arms by your side and palms facing in. Lift the weights so that your arms are parallel to the floor, and then raise both arms straight up over your head. Bring them both back down to the starting position and repeat. Keep abs firm and do not lock the elbow joint or lean backwards. Repeat x 15.

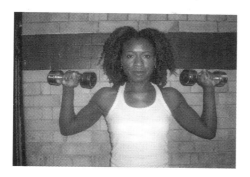 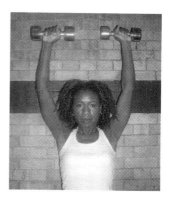

f) Bicep Curl: Sit straight and tall on the edge of a chair, with weights held in your hands, palms facing forward. Bring arms up to almost the top of your shoulders and then lower in a slow, controlled manner. Keep shoulders relaxed and chest open. Repeat x 15.

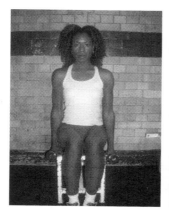 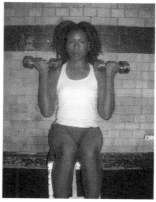

g) Triceps Dips: On a bench or chair placed up against a wall, reach behind your body and hold on to the edge with palms down, fingers forward; then slide your rear forward off the seat with feet hip-distance apart and knees bent. Bending at the elbow, lower your body toward the floor to produce a right angle, then push up with your arms. Repeat in a slow, controlled fashion x 15.

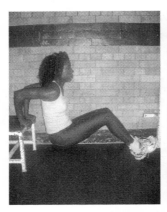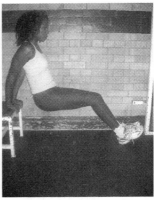

h) Pelvic Tilts:

Lie flat on your back on a mat or towel with your knees bent. Take a deep breath, then exhale, pulling your stomach in, and flatten your back into the floor. Hold this position for six seconds. Slowly release, breathe in and repeat (this is one rep). Do 20 reps.

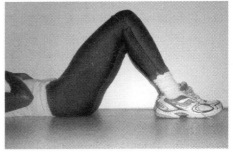

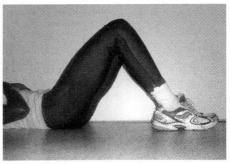

i) *Crunches:* Lie on your back with knees bent, feet hip-width apart and flat on the floor. Cross your arms in front of you with hands on opposite shoulders. Pull your stomach in and lift your head, neck, shoulder blades and chest up as one unit off the floor. As this is really a curling movement, make sure your chin remains down towards your chest. Exhale as you lift up, then slowly lower down to the floor and inhale. Repeat (this is one rep). Do 20 reps.

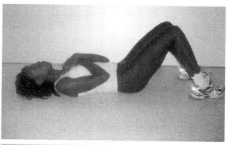
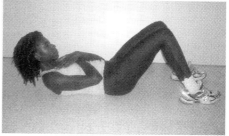

Programme B: Weeks 1–5

Cardio	5–10 mins bike warm-up
	20 mins stepper interval programme or treadmill manual programme power walk/jog (MHR 60–70 per cent)
	5 mins cool-down
Resistance	(Exercise instructions follow, below.)
Abs:	Crunches (hands in front/at side of head) – instructions below.
Stretches	Same as for Programme A

Exercise Instruction

Lie on the floor and adopt the Crunches position (above), only this time place your hands by either side of your head. Pull your stomach in and lift your head, neck, shoulder blades and chest up as one unit off the floor. Make sure you do not pull on your head or strain your neck. Repeat (this is one rep). Do 25 reps.

Programme A: Weeks 5–10

Cardio	5–10 mins bike warm-up
Cardio	5–10 mins bike or cross trainer warm-up
	20 mins jog/run on treadmill manual programme or stepper (MHR 70 per cent)
	3 mins cool-down
Resistance	(Exercise instructions follow, below.)
Legs:	Extension
	Curl
	Calf raises
	Gluteal raise
Chest:	Chest Press
Back:	Lat Pull-down
Shoulder:	Shoulder Press
Arms:	Bicep curl
	Triceps
Abs:	Ab roller – front curl
	Oblique Torso Twist
Stretches	Same as in weeks 1–5

Instructions: Weeks 5-10

a) *Extension:* Sit into the machine so that your back fits comfortably against the seat and the backs of your knees are at the edge of the padded seat. (This is an adjustable feature on most machines to suit members with different frames.) Adjust the weight stack to what you want to lift, then place the front of your feet under the padded roller. Slowly straighten your legs by bringing them upwards, until they are nearly parallel to the floor, then lower back to the starting position. Repeat x 15.

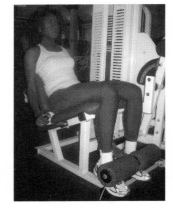

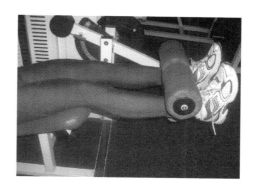

b) Curl: Lie face-down on the machine's bench, with your lower legs extending over the edge. Adjust the weight, then place your ankles under the padded rollers, holding on to the handles on each side of the bench. Slowly bring your heels towards your rear, keeping your hips pressed on to the bench and heels in contact with the roller. Lower gently to the starting position. Repeat x 15.

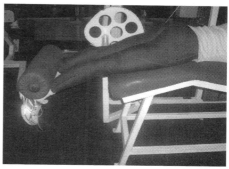

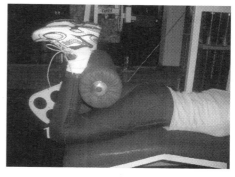

c) *Calf Raises:* Bend your knees to step on to the raised platform, with your shoulders comfortably under the pads and feet hip-distance apart, then stand up straight. Lift your body to the point where you are standing on your toes. Hold the contraction briefly, then slowly lower your heel to the starting position. Do not bounce, as the only movement should be at the ankle joint. Repeat x 15, but remember to bend your knees to move out of the machine.

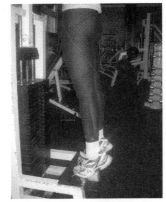

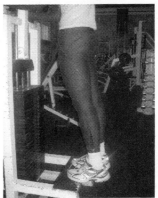

d) *Gluteal Raise:* Adjust the weight stack and sit into the machine so that your waist is anchored under the pads. Take a wide over-hand grip on the bar and pull it down to the front of your chest, just after the collar bone in a slow and controlled manner. Slowly return the bar to its starting

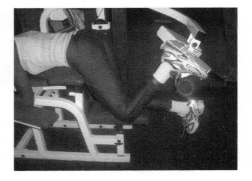

point and repeat (this is one rep). Do 10 reps.

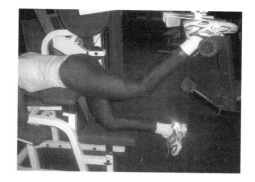

e) *Chest Press:* Depending on the machine's design, you may lie on your back and press the bar up or you sit in it upright. Make sure the handles are positioned at mid-point on the chest, and then press the bar away from your body, then lower. Keep your shoulders on the bench and elbows slightly bent. Repeat in a slow, controlled style (this is one rep). Do 15 reps.

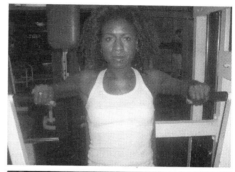

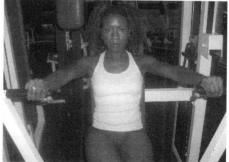

f) *Lat Pull-down:* Sit on the seat with your back to the weight stack, and press the bar up to an overhead position, without locking out the elbows. Keep your lower back on the back rest, then slowly lower the bar and repeat (this is one rep). Do 15 reps.

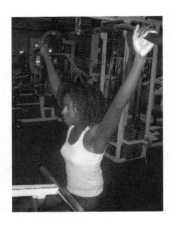
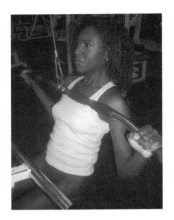

g) *Shoulder Press:* To begin, place your arms on the padded surface of the machine, ensuring that your shoulders and elbows form a line, then take hold of the handles with your palms facing up. Pull the handles towards your chin in an arc, lower slowly and repeat (this is one rep). Do 15 reps.

h) *Bicep Curl:* Stand in front of the machine, adjust the weight stack, then secure your feet under the pads. Lean back and take hold of the handles and sit down. In a slow and controlled manner, raise your hands towards your shoulders, keeping your elbows directly behind your body. Repeat (this is one rep). Do 15 reps.

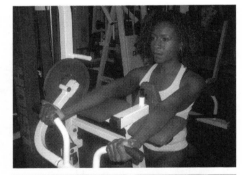
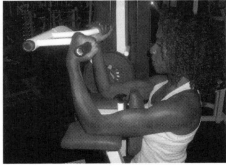

i) *Triceps:* Depending on the model of machine in front of you, either curl your legs under the padded bar or push up on a footpad at the back of the machine. Adjust the weight, then lift and lower the pad through a full range of motion and repeat (this is one rep). Do 15 reps.

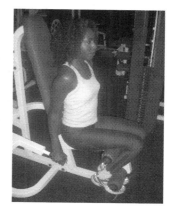

j) *Ab Roller:* Lie on the floor in the same position as you would for crunches. To start, place your head on the pads and your hands straight up, resting on the front of the machine. Tilt your pelvis up, then press on the bar and curl forward, so that your head, neck and shoulder blades are all off the floor. Slowly curl downwards, inhaling to the starting position, then repeat and exhale (this is one rep). Do 25 reps.

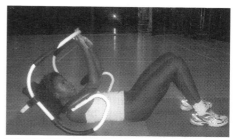

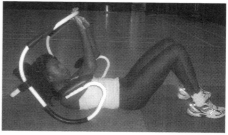

k) Oblique Torso Twist: Lie on the floor as you would for ordinary crunches but place your hands behind your head. Curl forward as you would in a crunch then, while lifted, rotate one shoulder towards the opposite knee. Do not pull with your elbow or twist your neck; just rotate your upper body. Think of bringing your shoulder to the opposite knee. Slowly, lower and repeat on the other side (this is one rep). Do 25 reps.

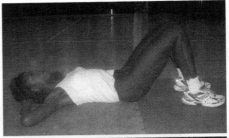

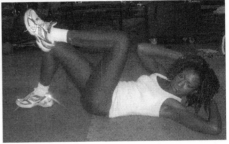

Programme B: Weeks 5–10

Cardio	5–10 mins bike warm-up
Cardio	30mins jog/run on treadmill hill programme level, or interval programme on the stepper (MHR 70–80 per cent)
Resistance	
Abs	Ball – instructions below.
Stretches	Same as in weeks 1–5

Exercise Instruction

Sit on a medium-sized ball with your toes touching the wall, lower back secured to the curve of the ball so that you are stable. Place your hands either side of your head and lift your torso as in your regular crunches, but lower your torso only to

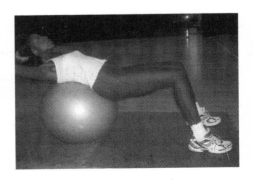

shoulder-blade height. Perform this move in a slow, controlled manner, keeping your shoulders relaxed and elbows pointing outwards throughout. Repeat x 25.

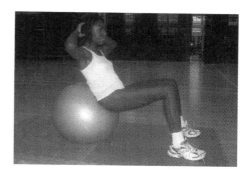

YOUR FUTURE

As an exercise practitioner it would have been easy for me simply to plug the benefits of exercise, but this would have been totally unsatisfactory and of little service to those truly wishing to move forward. In my view, daily holistic life practice is the only way to deal with the demands of the age we live in – a lifestyle such as this is by its very nature both preventative and the cure to the varied ailments that plague our lives.

The aim of this book has been to draw together two of the elements that most affect our everyday lives – health and wealth – in a way that helps us to see the reality behind our society's myth of abundance. Are we really a wealthy nation if thousands and millions of us suffer lives in pain, or indeed die from preventable illness? We have the opportunity to change this by taking a long-term view of how we can best maintain our bodies for the whole of our lives and not live solely for the pleasures of the present. This is one of the best wealth strategies you could make in your life. The whole health discussion needs to be positioned in a realistic socio-historical/economic environment rather than just blaming individuals. Not enough questions are being raised at a fundamental level about what motivates inactivity and unhealthy eating habits in the population.

Responsibility for our mass inertia has its roots in the fact that most of us have been ignorant about how our bodies work, and have destroyed many exercise facilities for political clout or financial gain. I hope that the results of such glaring short-sightedness can be corrected with more education and practical support in schools throughout Britain. Tools like those offered in this book help to redress this imbalance and offer an integrated health system.

Optimum health should be available to all, but I am not making wild promises of everlasting life, nor saying that you will never suffer illness or grow old. We should aspire to live and experience life in the best way we can – ailments like high blood pressure, heart disorders, obesity, osteoporosis and diabetes all devalue this experience. Choosing to reconnect with our bodies gives new meaning to each and every day.

Life expectancy figures constantly fluctuate – the only thing that is certain is that we will die. But the journey to that point is, to some extent, under our control if we are willing to take up the challenge of positively dealing with all the stimulation thrown at us. Eating healthily, exercising and using relaxation techniques help to reduce some of the physical and internal challenges of the journey, making us stronger in body and mind. It is this triad that sets up the integration for total and long-lasting health.

References

Introduction

1. http://news.bbc.co.uk/1/hi/in_depth/health/1420753.stm. See also Lee *et al.*, 'An examination of the impact of health and wealth depletion in elderly individuals', *J Gerontol B Psychol Sci Soc Sci* 2003 Mar; 58(2): S120-6

Chapter 1

1. E Guhl and W Koner, *The Greeks* (Senate,1994)
2. Richard Sennett, *Flesh and Stone* (Norton, 1976)
3. Norman Hampson, *The Enlightenment* (Penguin, 1982)

Chapter 3

1. Sarah Schenker, quoted in Philipps, Rachael, 'Science: Put a lid on it', *Independent* 31st January 1999

Chapter 4

1. Dr Ellen Billet, 'Phenylethylamine, a possible link to the antidepressant effects of exercise?', *British Journal of Sports Medicine* 2001; 35: 342-3
2. Dr J Blumenthal, 'Exercise can halt mental decline', *Journal of Ageing and Physical Activity*, January 2001
3. Dr Denise Park, 'Memories start failing in 20s', National Institute for Ageing, 2001; BBC on-line http://news.bbc.co.uk/1/hi/health/1490954.stm

Bibliography

American Council of Exercise, *Personal Trainer Manual* 1999 (http://www.acefitness.org/)

Anderson, Bob, *Stretching* (Pelham, 1981)

Andrews, John, 'Endurance', *Health and Fitness*, March 1992

Aristotle, *Ethics* (Penguin, 1976)

Atkins, Dr Robert, *New Diet Revolution* (Vermilion, 2003)

Baker, Emily, 'How to burn more calories', *Health and Fitness*, January 1995

Baker, Sue, 'New surveys reveal benefits of exercise on the mind', Mind Charity report, May 2001

Barker, Sarah, *The Alexander Technique* (Bantam, 1991)

Bartlett, S J and Mees, P D, 'Weight loss success', *Phys and Sports Med* 2001; 31(11)

Batman, Dr Paul, 'Resistance training and weight loss', *Fitness Network*, July 2003

Bee, Peta, 'Is this man obese?', *Sunday Times* 2001

Billet, Dr Ellen, 'Phenylethylamine, a possible link to the antidepressant effects of exercise?', *British Journal of Sports Medicine* 2001; 35: 342-3 (see also Billet, Dr Ellen, 'Why exercise cheers you up' – Nottingham Trent University September 2001 http://news.bbc.co.uk/1/hi/health/1565230.stm)

Blumenthal, Dr J, 'Exercise can halt mental decline', *Journal of Ageing and Physical Activity*, January 2001

Blythman, Joanna, 'Bite the Dust: pesticides in a healthy eater's shopping basket', *Observer* 10th May 2003

Boseley, Sarah, 'Particles of faith', *Guardian* 8th May 2004

Briffa, Dr John, 'Sweet Sorrow', *The Observer Magazine* 27th January 2002

------, 'Diet Plays a Role in Ovarian Cysts', *Observer* 16th November 2003

------, 'Midnight Munchers', *Observer* 8th February 2004

Carb Counter (Harper Collins, 2004)

Chaudhuri, Anita, 'Yoga, it's a rave', *Sunday Times* 28th September 2003

Chen, Joanne, 'Ab Fab – Good news: the six pack is officially passé', American *Vogue*, July 2002

Clarke, Jane, 'Stress busters', *Observer* 8th October 2000

Cochrane, Amanda, 'The Metabolic Rate', *Health and Fitness*, December 1991

Conway, D J, *Celtic Magic* (Llewellyn, 1991)

Cousins, David, *The Handbook for Light Workers* (Barton House, 1993)

Cox, Dr Richard, 'High-intensity exercise reduces stress and anxiety', *Research Quarterly for Exercise and Sport*, July 2003

Crespo, C J and Arbesman, J, 'Obesity in the United States', *Phys and Sports Med* 2003; 31(11)

Critser, Greg, 'Legacy of a Fat Man', *Guardian* 20th September 2003

Curry, Hazel, 'So will eating pasta after 5pm make you fat?', *Evening Standard* 20th May, 2003

D'Adamo, Dr Peter and Catherine Whitney, *Eat Right for Your Type* (Putnam, 1997)

------, *Live Right for Your Type* (Putnam, 2001)

Daly, Mary, *Gyn/Ecolgy* (The Women's Press, 1979)

Dobson, Rachel, 'Beyond Belief', *Sunday Times* 9th November 2003

Erasmus, Udo, *Fats That Heal, Fats That Kill* (Alive, 1998)

50+ Health, 'Activity and Health', www.50plushealth.co.uk April 2003

Fleckman, Douglas, 'The nature of stress and the mind–body connection', www.douglasfleckman.com

Fritjof, Capra, *The Web of Life* (Harper Collins, 1997)

Gawian, Shakti, *Creative Visualisation* (Nataraj, 2002)

Goodall, Jonathan, 'Drinking Yourself Fat', *Evening Standard* 21st May 2002

Griffin, Susan, *Women and Nature* (Harper and Row, 1978)

Guhl, E and Koner, W, *The Greeks* (Senate, 1994)

Hagan, Pat, 'Body signs that reveal the strain', *Evening Standard* March 2004

Hampson, Norman, *The Enlightenment* (Penguin, 1982)

Heart UK, 'Heart Health', *Sunday Times* March 2003

Hobsbawn, E J, *The Age of Revolution* (Abacus, 1986)

Holford, Patrick, *Optimum Nutrition Bible* (Piatkus, 1998)

Intelligent Fitness, 'Fat Loss: The Science of Assessment, Nutrition and Exercise Prescription', June 2003

Jarvie, Catherine, 'Fighting with Food' *Observer* 19th October 2003

Kenton, Leslie, *The X Factor Diet* (Vermilion, 2002)

Lawrence, Felicity, 'Miles and miles and miles: How far has your basket of food travelled?', *Guardian* 10th May 2003

------, *Not on the Label* (Penguin, 2004)

Lee *et al.*, 'An examination of the impact of health and wealth depletion in elderly individuals', *J Gerontol B Psychol Sci Soc Sci* 2003 Mar; 58(2): S120-6

Leeds, Dr Antony and Miller, Jennie, *The GI Factor* (Hodder and Stoughton, 1996)

Leith, William, 'Who can we trust in the Atkins backlash?', *Evening Standard* January 2004

Le Shan, Lawrence, *How to Meditate* (Bantam, 1982)

Lycholat, Tony, 'Resistance training for healthy adults', *Fit Pro* magazine 1998; www.fitpro.com

McKeith, Gillian, *Living Food for Health* (Piatkus, 2000)

McKie, Robin, 'Praise the Lard', *Observer* 11th August 2002

Macnair, Dr Trisha, 'Stress can rot the brain', *British Medical Journal* 1997; 315: 530–35

Marber, Ian, 'Are these foods making you ill?', *Evening Standard* 15th May 2001

Mindell, Earl, *Earl Mindell's New Vitamin Bible* (Souvenir Press, 2005)

Mitchell, Emma, 'Wellbeing, nutritional value of our food today', *Guardian* September 2003

Murphy, Sam, 'Let's get physical', *Guardian* February 2003

------, 'Labouring under falsehoods', *Guardian* September 2003

Myss, Caroline, *Anatomy of the Spirit* (Bantam, 1997)

O'Neil, Matt, 'Meal Timing for weight loss', *Fit Pro* February 2004; www.fitpro.com

Oakeshott, Isabel, 'Counting Calories is a waste of time', *Evening Standard* November 2003

Paine, Andre, 'They're young, professional and tired by 35', *Evening Standard* September 2003

Park, Dr Denise, 'Memories start failing in 20s', National Institute for Ageing US August 2001; BBC on-line http://news.bbc.co.uk/1/hi/health/1490954.stm

Parry, Robert, *Teach Yourself Tai Chi* (McGraw-Hill, 2001)

Pearson, Martin, 'Antioxidants', *Health and Fitness*, May 1995

Philipps, Rachael, 'Science: Put a lid on it', *Independent* 31st January 1999

Redfield, James, *The Celestine Prophecy* (Bantam, 1994)

Rendel, Peter, *Understanding the Chakras* (Aquarian, 1990)

Revill, Jo, 'A Deadly Slice of American Pie', *Observer* 21st September 2003

------, 'Official: Atkins diet can be deadly', *Observer* 21st September 2003

------, 'Life makes you sick', *Observer* 12th October 2003

------, 'Binge drinking: do they mean us?' *Observer* December 2003

Sennett, Richard, *Flesh and Stone* (Norton, 1976)

Shealy, Norman *et al.*, *The Complete Encyclopaedia of Natural Healing Therapies* (Element, 1999)

Sinatra, Dr Stephen, *Lower Your Blood Pressure* (Piatkus, 2003)

Stairmaster, *The Fitness Handbook* (2nd edn; 1995)

Stewart, Marion, *The Phyto Factor* (Vermilion, 2000)

University of Iowa, 'Stress and its Effects on the body', www.uihealthcare.com

Ursell, Amanda, 'How to Eat', *Sunday Times* July 2003

------, 'Trans-fats', *Sunday Times* March 2004

Wescott, Wayne *et al.*, 'Back to basics', *Fit Pro* 1996; www.fitpro.com

Which Report, 'Water Consumption', October 2000

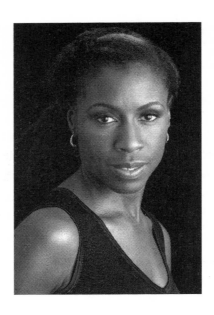

For more than 15 years, Jacqueline Harvey has created and taught holistic personal fitness programmes that help clients achieve their weight goals, increase their fitness levels and improve their total health profile. By using an integrated approach, Jacqueline's programmes help anyone who genuinely wants to improve the quality of their life. Following her research into both Western and Eastern philosophies/life-systems she has built health and fitness programmes that really get results.

In 2005, she set up a premium-quality health-management service called 'Crystal Clear Health' – her team of practitioners offer intensive solutions to lifestyle-generated health problems.

Based at the Jubilee Hall Fitness Club in London's Covent Garden, Jacqueline's clients include many successful business people and celebrities – Erin O'Connor, Kate Silverton, Brenda Emmanus and Fearne Cotton.

Since 1997, Jacqueline has been the feature health writer for *The Singer* magazine, contributing interviews, restaurant reviews and previews of new shows both nationally and internationally. She has contributed to *Health and Fitness* and *Don't Tell It* magazines with features on health/fitness issues, and more recently has written for *Colures* magazine.

As a broadcast presenter, Jacqueline has fronted health and fitness on television, radio and for fitness brands such as Nike, Gossards – Shock Absorber and Khaya yoga wear. In addition, she has also presented her Lighten Up workshops for corporations and The Pascal Theatre Company both in London and throughout the UK.

Passionate about health, fitness and food, Jacqueline enjoys London's culture, be it dining out, singing gospel and jazz music, visiting art exhibitions, going to the cinema or occasionally relaxing at home with music and a good book.

Titles of Related Interest

YOU CAN HEAL YOUR LIFE, the movie, starring Louise L. Hay & Friends
(available as a 1-DVD set and an expanded 2-DVD set)
Watch the trailer at **www.LouiseHayMovie.com**

The True You Diet, by Dr John Briffa
Everything I've Done That Worked, by Lesley Garner
Time Management for Manic Mums, by Allison Mitchell
You Can Heal Your Life, by Louise L. Hay
The Healing Power of Nature Foods, by Susan Smith Jones
You Can Have What You Want, by Michael Neill